Praises for Bragg Healthy Lifestyle and the Bragg Healthy Heart Book

These are just a few of the thousands of testimonials we receive yearly, praising The Bragg Health Books for the Super Health and rejuvenation benefits they reap – physically, mentally and spiritually. We also look forward to hearing from you soon.

When I was a young gymnastics coach at Stanford University, Paul Bragg's words and example inspired me to live a healthy lifestyle. I was twenty-three then; now I am over 63, and my health serves as a living testimonial to Bragg's health wisdom, carried on by his dedicated health crusading daughter, Patricia. Thank you!
– Dan Millman, author *The Way of the Peaceful Warrior*
• *www.peacefulwarrior.com*

Paul Bragg saved my life when I attended Bragg Health Crusade in Oakland. At 15 I was so weak and sickly, that I had to wear a back brace to sit up. I thank Bragg Healthy Lifestyle for my long, healthy, active life and I love spreading health and fitness.
– Jack LaLanne, Bragg follower and Fitness Pioneer to 97
• *www.JackLalanne.com*

As a youth I had a learning disability and was told I would never read, write or communicate normally. At 14 I dropped out of school and at 17 ended up in Hawaii surfing. My road to recovery led me to Paul Bragg who changed my life by giving me one simple affirmation to repeat: "I am a genius and I apply my wisdom." Paul Bragg inspired me to go back to school and get my education and from there miracles happened. I have authored 72 training programs and 40 books and love to crusade around the world thanks to Paul Bragg. – Dr. John Demartini, Dynamic Crusader Star in *The Secret* • *www.DrDemartini.com*

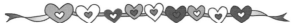

As I stride along on my daily 3-4 mile brisk walk that helps me maintain a healthier heart, body and keeps my bones strong, I say to myself, often out loud, "Health, Strength, Youth, Vitality, Joy, Peace and Salvation for Eternity!"
– Patricia Bragg, Health Crusader

A

Praises for Bragg Healthy Lifestyle and the Bragg Healthy Heart Book

Thank you Paul and Patricia Bragg for my simple, easy to follow Bragg Healthy Lifestyle. You make my days healthy!
– Clint Eastwood, Academy Award Winning Film Producer, Director, actor and Bragg follower for over 60 years

In Medical School I read Dr. Bragg's Health Books. They changed my way of thinking and the path of my life. I founded Omega Institute.
– Stephan Rechtschaffen, M.D. • www.eOmega.org

Thanks to Paul Bragg and Bragg Books, my childhood asthma was cured in one month with Bragg Healthy Lifestyle Living.
– Paul Wenner, creator of the Gardenburger

Thanks to the Bragg Health Books, they were our introduction to healthy living. We are very grateful to you and your father.
– Marilyn Diamond, co-author, *Fit For Life* Best-Seller 40 weeks

Paul Bragg inspired me many years ago with the "Miracle of Fasting" and with his philosophy on health. His daughter Patricia is a testament to the ageless value of living the Bragg Healthy Lifestyle. – Jay Robb, author *The Fruit Flush*

I have known the Bragg Health Books over 30 years. They are a blessing to me and my family and to all who read them to help make this a healthier world. – Pastor Mike MacIntosh, Horizon Christian Fellowship, San Diego, CA

Thanks to Bragg *Miracle of Fasting* and *Healthy Lifestyle* books, we're healthy, fit and singing better and staying younger than ever!
– The Beach Boys • www.TheBeachBoys.com

I am following the Bragg Healthy Lifestyle which I heard of through a friend. Your books are motivators and have blessed my health and life and are making perfect gifts for my family and friends. – Delphine, Singapore

Bragg Books were my conversion to the healthy way.
– James Balch, M.D., co-author of
Prescription for Nutritional Healing

B

Praises for Bragg Healthy Lifestyle and the Bragg Healthy Heart Book

I love the Bragg Books, especially *The Miracle of Fasting*. They are so popular and loved in Russia and the Ukraine. I give thanks for my health and my super energy. I won the famous Honolulu Marathon with the all-time women's record! – Lyubov Morgunova, Champion Runner, Moscow, Russia

Thank you Patricia for our first meeting in London in 1968. When I was feeling my years, you gave me your *Miracle of Fasting* Book – it got me exercising – doing brisk walking and eating more wisely. You were a blessing God-sent and just when I needed to get more healthily recharged for Crusading. – Reverend Billy Graham • *www.BillyGraham.org*

Thanks to you and your wonderful father for your guidance and teaching over the years. What a great gift you and your father have provided for us all through your Bragg Health Books and wonderful Bragg Health Products. Your Fasting and Vinegar books have improved my life immensely. I've lost 30 lbs. and feel years younger. At 67 youthful years, I give thanks for the great benefits of health I enjoy because of the work you and your father have so generously dedicated your lives too!! Wishing you every blessing under the Sun. – Captain Wes Herman (retired) Santa Barbara County Fire Dept.

Your dad, Dr. Paul Bragg IS the FATHER of the natural health industry and the entire natural health movement. Everything that has been done in natural health and physical culture since has been based on the pioneering vision and principles articulated by Dr. Bragg. He gave us all our health direction! – Dr. William Wong

I thank Paul Bragg for his Health Pioneering and Crusading. Dr. Bragg paved the way for our 100% healthy principles and inspired me to start Good Earth Restaurants. I am a Bragg Product user and enthusiast. – Bill Galt, CA

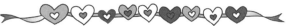

Happiness is when . . . what you think, what you say, how you live, and what you do are in peaceful harmony. – Mahatma Gandhi

C

Praises for Bragg Healthy Lifestyle and the Bragg Healthy Heart Book

In 1975 I was diagnosed with coronary heart disease. I followed the Free Bragg Exercise Classes and Health Lectures at Fort DeRussy lawn, Waikiki Beach, 6 days a week. Years have passed and I am going strong and healthy, thanks to The Bragg Healthy Lifestyle. In 1930's my father had severe hip arthritis and hardly able to walk. He followed the Bragg Healthy Lifestyle, and daily made his vinegar drink.
– Helen Risk, RN, Hawaii

The Bragg Healthy Lifestyle with Fasting has changed my life! I lost weight and my energy levels went through the roof. I look forward to "Fasting" days. I think better and I am a better husband and father. Thank you Patricia, this has been a great blessing in my life. Also, thank you for sharing the Bragg Healthy Lifestyle at our "AOL" Conference.
– Byron H. Elton, VP Entertainment, Time Warner AOL

I give thanks to Health Crusaders Paul Bragg and daughter Patricia for their dedicated years of service spreading health as our Lord wants us healthy! It's made a great difference in my life and millions worldwide. – Pat Robertson, Host CBN "700" Club

I'd like to thank you for teaching me how to take control of my health! I have lost 55 pounds. I feel "Great!" Bragg books have showed me vitality, happiness and being close to Mother Nature. You are real "Crusaders of Health." – Leonard Amato

Dear Friends – you can not know how greatly you have already impacted my life and many of my friends and family! We love your Bragg Health Books, teachings and products, and we are now living healthier, happier lives. Thank You!
– Winnie Brown, Arizona

I am a big fan of Paul Bragg. I fast follow the Bragg Healthy Lifestyle daily. The world and I are blessed with the health teachings of Paul and Patricia Bragg!
– Anthony "Tony" Robbins • www.AnthonyRobbins.com

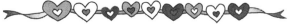

A laugh is just like sunshine, it freshens all the day. – Heart Warmers

Praises for Bragg Healthy Lifestyle and the Bragg Healthy Heart Book

It was in Hawaii when I began to realize that while lifestyle choices can not only be a major negative to health and well-being, but lifestyle can be a winning asset to wellness! My discovery on fitness and health began shortly after I arrived in Hawaii at age 19 when I discovered Paul Bragg, the great health and fitness pioneer teaching a free exercise class 6 days a week at Waikiki Beach.
– Kathy Smith, Hollywood, CA • *www.KathySmith.com*

I had the opportunity to sit next to Patricia on a flight from Dallas to L.A. Her honesty about my weight and health really inspired me to make great improving life changes! A year later, I am 85 lbs. lighter and heart rate cut almost in half. Patricia you helped save my life! – Mike Ableman, Texas

In the past our family has had chronic health problems. Within the last year and a half God has shown us His Will for healing and divine health. Our journey has included a healthy diet, some fasting and a complete change in lifestyle. We tried ACV and I want you to know that it is one of the most valuable changes that we have included in our lifestyle! It is terrific! I cannot express how good we feel! I am so thankful for every good thing that God has put before us – this journey, and every miraculous result and ACV is part of that. Thank you for sharing this wealth of health in Bragg Books. God Bless You! – Rhonda Jackson, Oklahoma

I was diagnosed with diabetes and had high sugar levels. After following Bragg Healthy Lifestyle for 6 months, now I am insulin free and healthier than I have been for the last 15 years. My wife, three children and I are now healthy vegetarians living the Bragg Healthy Lifestyle. Results have been amazing. We thank You.
– Dennis Urbans, Australia

For over 40 years I've followed Bragg Healthy Lifestyle – it teaches you how to take control of your health and build a healthy future.
– Mark Victor Hansen, co-creator, *Chicken Soup for Soul* Series

Good health and good sense are two of life's greatest blessings.
– Publilius Syrus, Latin Writer, 42 B.C.

E

Praises for Bragg Healthy Lifestyle and the Bragg Healthy Heart Book

Patricia Bragg is a dedicated Health Crusader and she shared her Bragg Healthy Lifestyle with millions of our radio listeners. Thank you Patricia.
– Host George Noory, Coast to Coast Radio

How did I beat cancer, obesity, diabetes, strep, three herniated disks and excruciating pain? The answer was changing to the Bragg's Healthy Lifestyle and having the amazing vinegar drink daily. It changed my life and I also lost 70 lbs! I received a new life and that is just the beginning because my manhood returned that was lost to diabetes – now that's exciting! On my trip to Honolulu I visited the famous free Bragg Exercise Class at Waikiki Beach. I became so regenerated with a wonderful new viewpoint towards living the Bragg Healthy Lifestyle that I now live in Hawaii. I'm invigorated with new energy for life and living! My new purpose for living is to help others reclaim their health rights! I want the world to join The Bragg Health Crusade. I am so thankful to Paul and Patricia for being my inspiration. – Len, Hawaii

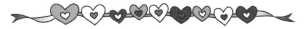

We get letters daily at our Santa Barbara headquarters. We would love to receive a testimonial letter from you on any blessings, healings and changes you experienced after following The Bragg Healthy Lifestyle and this book. It's all within your grasp to be in top health. By following this book, you can reap more Super Health and a happy, longer vital life! It's never too late to begin. Studies show amazing results that were obtained by exercise with people even in their 80's and 90's – pages 106 to 107. You can receive miracles with healthy nutrition, fasting and exercise! Start now!

Daily our prayers & love go out to you, your heart, mind & soul with love.

Patricia Bragg

3 John 2

Miracles can happen every day through guidance and prayer! – Patricia Bragg

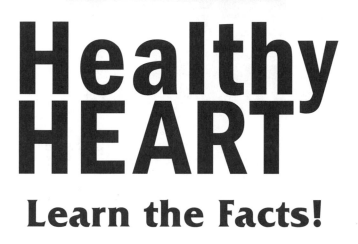

Patricia Bragg Books

Healthy HEART

Learn the Facts!

Support Your Cardiovascular System At Any Age

PAUL C. BRAGG, N.D., Ph.D.
LIFE EXTENSION SPECIALIST

and

PATRICIA BRAGG
HEALTH CRUSADER & LIFESTYLE EDUCATOR

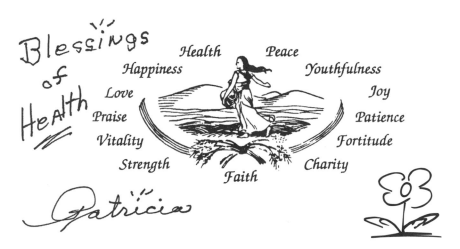

Blessings of Health

Health   Peace
Happiness   Youthfulness
Love   Joy
Praise   Patience
Vitality   Fortitude
Strength   Charity
Faith

Patricia

BECOME
A Health Crusader – for a 100% Healthy World for All!

www.PatriciaBraggBooks.com

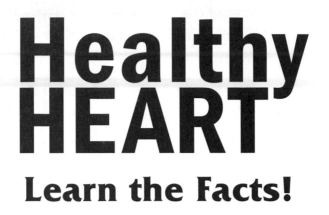

Healthy HEART

Learn the Facts!

Support Your Cardiovascular System At Any Age

PAUL C. BRAGG, N.D., Ph.D.
LIFE EXTENSION SPECIALIST
and
PATRICIA BRAGG
HEALTH CRUSADER & LIFESTYLE EDUCATOR

Visit our website:
www.PatriciaBraggBooks.com

Eighteenth Edition MMXXI
ISBN: 978-0-87790-081-8

Library of Congress Cataloging-in-Publication Data on file with publisher

Published in the United States
HEALTH SCIENCE
7127 Hollister Avenue, Suite 25A, Box 249, Santa Barbara, CA 93117
Toll-Free: (833) 408-1122

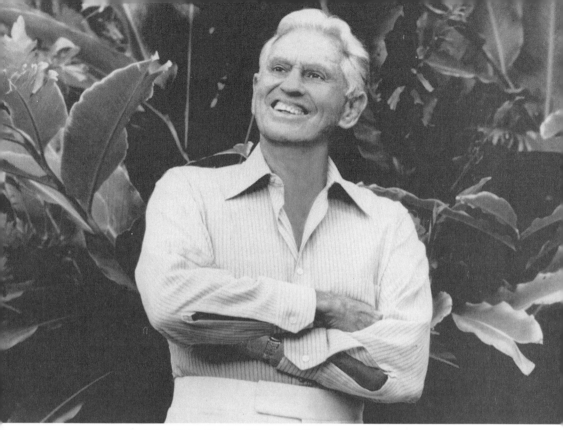

PAUL C. BRAGG, N.D., Ph.D.
World's Leading Healthy Lifestyle Authority

Paul C. Bragg's daughter Patricia and their wonderful, healthy members of the Bragg *Longer Life, Health and Happiness Club* exercised daily on the beautiful Fort DeRussy lawn, at famous Waikiki Beach in Honolulu, Hawaii. On Saturday there were often health lectures on how to live a long, healthy life! The group averaged 50 to 75 per day, depending on the season. From December to March it can go up to 125. Its dedicated leaders carried on the class for over 43 years. Thousands visited the club from around the world and carried the Bragg Health and Fitness Crusade to friends and relatives back home.

Your body is a non-stop living system, in constant motion 24 hours daily, cleaning, repairing, healing and growing. – Patricia Bragg

To maintain good health, normal weight and increase the good life of radiant health, joy and happiness, the body must be exercised properly (stretching, walking, jogging, biking, swimming, deep breathing, good posture) and nourished with healthy foods. – Paul C. Bragg, N.D., Ph.D.

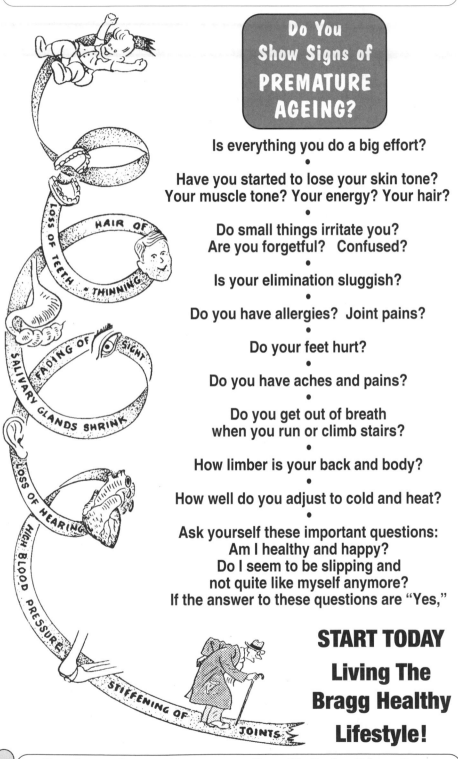

Do You Show Signs of PREMATURE AGEING?

Is everything you do a big effort?

Have you started to lose your skin tone?
Your muscle tone? Your energy? Your hair?

Do small things irritate you?
Are you forgetful?   Confused?

Is your elimination sluggish?

Do you have allergies? Joint pains?

Do your feet hurt?

Do you have aches and pains?

Do you get out of breath
when you run or climb stairs?

How limber is your back and body?

How well do you adjust to cold and heat?

Ask yourself these important questions:
Am I healthy and happy?
Do I seem to be slipping and
not quite like myself anymore?
If the answer to these questions are "Yes,"

START TODAY
Living The
Bragg Healthy
Lifestyle!

He who understands nature walks with God. – Edgar Cayce

Why My Father & I Wrote This Heart Book:

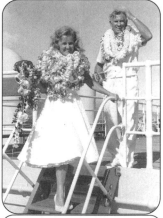

World Health Crusaders
Paul C. Bragg and
daughter Patricia

Cardiovascular (heart and blood vessel) problems constitute the #1 Killer in the civilized world today. Yet these deadly problems can be prevented, controlled and even reversed! Millions of our health students around the world have developed strong hearts from weak hearts. Many have averted heart surgery and helped their health and their heart by living this Bragg Healthy Lifestyle and Heart Program.

My father, Paul C. Bragg, pioneered these precepts and practiced them diligently with an "ageless" heart in a biologically youthful body even as a great-great-grandfather! We have both thrived on our diet of healthy natural foods. No salt, no refined white sugar or flour, no artificial additives or poisonous preservatives, no debilitating drinks, only natural "live" foods, fresh organic fruits and vegetables and their juices and distilled water combined with a program of healthful exercise, fasting, relaxation and revitalizing sleep.

We want to share with you the knowledge we have gained from our years of combined experience and research so you may no longer fear and dread this #1 Killer. Choose to be healthy and fit and remain young in heart for your entire life! It's up to you!

 Bragg Healthy Lifestyle Plan

- *Read, plan, plot, and follow through for supreme health and longevity.*
- *Underline, highlight or dog-ear pages as you read important passages.*
- *Organizing your lifestyle helps you identify what's important in your life.*
- *Be faithful to your health goals everyday for a healthy, long, happy life.*
- *Where space allows we have included 'words of wisdom' from great minds to motivate and inspire you. Please share your favorite sayings with us.*
- *Write us about your successes following The Bragg Healthy Lifestyle.*

May you be healthy all the days of your life. – Jonathan Swift, 1745

A book is a garden, an orchard, a storehouse, a party, a mentor and teacher.
Books can be your guideposts and faithful counsellors. – Henry Ward Beecher

---

Bragg Health Books are here to guide you to Super Health!

✿ Cautionary Note and Disclaimer ✿

The information provided here is for educational purposes only. Any decision on your part to read, listen and use this information is your personal choice. The information in this book is not meant to be used to diagnose, prescribe or treat any illness. Please discuss any changes you wish to make to your medical treatment with a qualified, licensed health care provider.

If you are taking medication to control your blood sugar or blood pressure, you may need to reduce the dosage if you significantly restrict your carbohydrate intake. This is best done under the care and supervision of an experienced and qualified licensed health care provider. Anyone who has any other serious illness such as cardiovascular disease, cancer, kidney or liver disease needs to exercise caution if making dietary changes. You should consult your physician for guidance. If you are pregnant or lactating, you should not overly restrict protein or fat intake. Also, young children and teens have much more demanding nutrient needs and should NOT have their protein or fat intake overly restricted.

The information presented in this book is in no way intended as medical advice or a substitute for medical counseling. It is intended only to provide the opinions and ideas of the authors. It is sold with the understanding that the authors are not engaged in rendering medical, health or any other kind of professional services in this book. The reader should consult his or her medical doctor, or any other competent professional, before adopting any of the suggestions in this book, or drawing inferences from it.

The authors disclaim any responsibility for any liability, loss or risk, personal or otherwise, which is incurred as a consequence, directly or indirectly, of the use and application of the contents of this book.

Please consult your physician before beginning this program, and use all of the information the authors suggest in conjunction with the guidance and care of your physician. Your physician should be aware of all medical conditions that you may have, as well as medications and supplements you are taking.

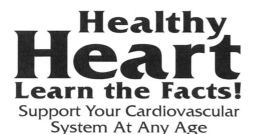

Healthy Heart
Learn the Facts!
Support Your Cardiovascular System At Any Age

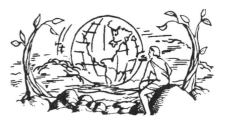

To preserve health is a moral and religious duty, for health is the basis for all social virtues. We can no longer be as useful when not well.
– Dr. Samuel Johnson, Father of Dictionaries, 1755

Contents

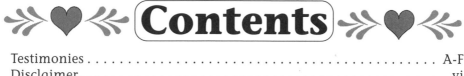

Bragg Books are silent, faithful, health teachers – never tiring, ready night or day to help you help yourself to health!

Life is learning which rules to obey and which rules not to obey and the wisdom to tell the difference between the two!

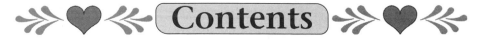

Contents

*Talk happiness! Talk faith! Live healthy! Say you are well, and all is
well with you, and God shall hear your words and make them true.*
– Ella Wheeler-Wilcox

*Living in harmony with the universe is living totally alive, full of vitality,
health, joy, power, love, and abundance on every level. – Shakti Gawain*

*Kindness should be a frame of mind in which we are alert to every chance:
to do, to improve, to give, to share and to cheer. – Patricia Bragg*

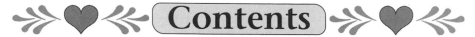

Contents

Progress is impossible without change, and those who cannot
change their minds, cannot change anything! – George Bernard Shaw

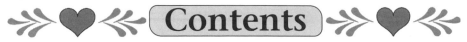

Contents

Contents

This Heart Book guides you to have a stronger, healthier, younger heart!

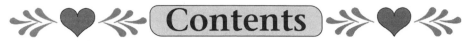

Contents

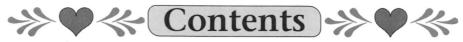

Contents

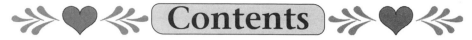

Contents

Practice politeness, it goes far, yet costs you nothing. – Seneca

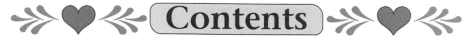

Contents

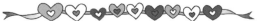

Love doesn't make the world go round.
Love is what makes the ride more worthwhile. – F. P. Jones

Contents

Three Needed Health Habits

*There are 3 habits which, with but one condition added, will give you every
thing in the world worth having, beyond which the imagination of man cannot
conjure forth a single additional improvement! These habits are:*

- **The Health Habit** - **The Work Habit** - **The Study Habit**

*If you have these habits, and also have the love of someone who has these
same habits, you are both in paradise now and here. – Elbert Hubbard*

*If I were to name the three most precious resources of life, I would say books,
friends and nature; and the greatest of these, at least the most constant and
always at hand is Mother Nature and God. – John Burroughs*

*When health is absent, wisdom cannot reveal itself,
art can't manifest, strength can't fight, wealth becomes useless,
and intelligence can't be applied. – Herophilus*

*You can personally significantly decrease the odds of having a heart attack.
It requires improving eating and exercising habits. We guide you in this book.*

*The better informed you are, the more committed you'll be to making the
changes necessary to lower your chances of having a heart attack or stroke.*

*The more natural food you eat, the more you'll enjoy radiant health and
be able to promote the higher life of love and brotherhood. – Patricia Bragg*

Chapter 1

Your Precious Body
And the Body's Miraculous
Life Pump – Your Heart

Suppose a magician suddenly appeared before you and promised you a marvelous machine which could run itself, direct itself, repair itself and perform remarkable mental and physical feats. Would you treasure such a machine? Of course you would! You would keep it in top condition in order to obtain and enjoy a maximum of service. Daily you would be astonished anew by the performance of this miracle-machine!

True, this is an age of computers, biotechnology and other modern mechanical, scientific and outer space marvels. Remember that the supreme tribute we can pay to any machine is to say, *It is almost human.* Now, stop and think! Mother Nature has presented you with the world's most miraculous machine – your own body! This incredible factory has its own *non-stop motor* (the heart), its own *fueling system* (the digestive system), its own human *filtration system* (the kidneys), its own *thinking computer* (brain and nervous system), and its own *temperature controls* (sweat glands), etc. Indeed, this miraculous creation even has the *power to reproduce* itself!

Keep Your Precious Body and Your Heart Functioning at Peak Efficiency

Despite its importance, most of us rarely consider the care of this machine – our body – until illness strikes. By *care* we don't mean *coddling*. Instead, we mean those sensible practices and precautions which keep us in shape for the vigorous daily routine that strenuous modern living requires. Most people are fortunate to be born healthy, but far too often take this priceless gift of health for granted. Unfortunately, Mother Nature does not always let them get away with this carefree attitude. You can ruin a good car by neglect or abuse, and you can do the same with your heart and body!

Unless you know how your body functions or malfunctions, it's difficult to take proper care of it. Most people's ideas about their physical processes are erroneous or far-fetched. Even in this scientific age, too many superstitions and misconceptions about the human body still persist.

In this book we will explain how the body works, with a straightforward account of the physical, mental and emotional factors which influence it. There will be valuable suggestions on how to keep your heart, brain, body and its entire system running at peak efficiency.

Don't Blame Heart Attacks on Hard Work, Stress, Strain or Tension

You hear a great deal about the modern *rat race* today. You hear people saying that our *mile-a-minute* pace of living causes heart attacks. The words *hard work*, *stress* and *tension* are excuses for rising heart attack death rates. (Reread Healthy Heart Habits on inside front cover.)

The basis for a heart attack is coronary blockage! The question is often asked, *Is there no warning before the blood supply to the heart begins to get dangerously low?* The answer is simple: arterial blockage grows silently and insidiously! There is usually no way of knowing exactly how much and where plaque is accumulating inside one's arteries, usually until it's too late.

In some parts of the body, such as the legs, a reduced blood supply to the muscles can cause localized pain and cramping sensations! The heart sometimes gives angina pain warnings (page 17). Often there's no pain warning. This is why so many people will tell you they are in fine shape (no pain, problems, etc.) without taking special care of their bodies. Unfortunately, many are potentially killing themselves with their unhealthy lifestyle. When the heart attack comes, do they ever blame it on unhealthy habits? Oh, no! They blame hard work, pressures and tensions!

Unhealthy cooking diminishes happiness and shortens life. – Wisdom of Ages

The Lord gives rest and strength to those who are weary. – Isaiah 40:29

Primitive Humans Lived and Thrived Under Great Pressures

Let's set the record straight: humans have lived under tremendous pressure, stress, strain and tension since the dawn of history. That is what life partly is – a struggle! To live is to exist under pressures of all kinds. Humans have never lived without some challenges – even today!

In order to survive, our primitive ancestors lived under pressures that would be difficult for us to handle in today's modern world. Early humans were often the prey of wild animals seeking to kill them. Wind, rain, snow and bad weather would also put them under severe duress. Humans had to survive cruel natural calamities like floods, tornadoes, earthquakes, hurricanes, plagues, famines and epidemics. In short, stress and tension are nothing new to humanity. Therefore, we believe humans can face and overcome almost all of the hardest pressures life puts upon them if they are healthy, strong of body and alert of mind.

The Secret of Survival

Heart trouble need not be an inevitable by-product of mounting work, stress, tension and pressures that people face daily. Though early generations had to exist under tremendous pressure, they were rugged; active physically and mentally. Their secret was simple living, natural foods (without preservatives and pesticides) and ample pure air as well as hard work, which exercises and tones the heart and muscles. As it was in the past, so it is today. Build yourself a vigorous, strong body so that you may face the great pressures of our culture today! Health, strength, endurance, stamina, vitality and energy are your protection from pressure, stress, strain and tension!

Exercise reduces the risk of heart disease through direct effects on your cardiovascular system and through reduction of intra-abdominal stomach fat.
 The health goal of exercise and maintaining normal weight is to lower the potential for cardiovascular disease.
– American Heart Association (see pages 18 and 246)

Develop healthy self-esteem to generate positive lifestyle habits that will promote more serenity, peace and love in your life. – Patricia Bragg

Self-Preservation is the First Law of Life

This book is about having a healthy and fit heart and body. All of us must get fit for the long battle of life! There is no substitute for living a healthy life. It's up to you, whether you're rich or poor, to fight for your health and longevity with healthy eating and ample exercise!

Hundreds of times we have heard wealthy people say, *I'd give all my wealth for my health!* If they had applied a combination of common sense and a little effort, they easily could have had both! All that is necessary is an elementary knowledge of the workings of the body and its basic needs, combined with the ability to recognize abuse and the willpower to avoid it! People spend years mastering their careers. However, devoting minutes daily learning about the health needs and limitations of their bodies seems difficult for them. **Most people tend to ignore the fact that enjoying well-earned prosperity and long, happy lives depends on their health!**

You Can Restore Your Health and Your Heart

One of the most remarkable miracles about the human body is its ability to repair and heal itself! For example, if you cut yourself, your body heals the cut. If you break a bone, the body heals the bone after it's set and often it becomes stronger than before. Unexpected injury may happen at any time and to *anyone*! However, if you have been taking care of your body, chances are you will recover more quickly and with less discomfort.

The less obvious injuries that we accumulate over time may also be repaired by the amazing human body. After taking a hammering for years, after being totally neglected for too long, *your body can experience astounding recovery and rejuvenation!* You must be prepared to be patient and generous with your time and effort. Just as a business that has been allowed to slip, can be rebuilt, so can a neglected body! (See Conrad Hilton Story, page 201.) Don't expect a miracle overnight – *Rome wasn't built in a day*. It takes time and dedication to rebuild broken health.

Your heart takes care of you and keeps you alive, please be good to it!
– Paul C. Bragg, Originator of Health Food Stores

Coronary Disease is Preventable & Reversible

Dr. Dean Ornish's book *Reversing Heart Disease* states: *Heart problems are not only preventable, but also reversible by changing your lifestyle.* (See web: *www.Ornish.com*) We agree – if people would only eat and exercise properly, coronary disease could be stopped in its tracks! Future heart problems would be prevented and heart disease would begin to reverse! People have the power in their own mind to take control of their lives! Many people never know physical super health. They miss out on the priceless benefits of living The Bragg Healthy Lifestyle.

An Ounce of Prevention is Worth A Ton of Cure Towards Your Building an Ageless Heart

Living by The Bragg Healthy Lifestyle principles of proper diet, ample exercise, plenty of rest, and deep breathing, promotes supreme health and longevity. Most people wait until something bad happens to their body before they do anything. We will teach you how to care for your body, so you can have a healthy and powerful heart at any age! Start today – it's priceless, exciting and fun! Challenge yourself – you will rebuild not only your heart, but your entire body!

The Bragg Healthy Lifestyle begins with nutrition. We obtain most of our energy from the food we eat, which has been directly or indirectly acted upon by the rays of the sun. Therefore, a *healthy diet* is important for the creation and maintenance of health. We must not only eat correctly, but also drink the right fluids. Pure distilled water is essential. The next crucial step is keeping oxygen-rich healthy blood circulating throughout the body's great blood pipe system. This is accomplished with daily vigorous exercise and activity. The results will be worth all the effort you put into improving your diet and exercise. Your rewards will be a more powerful heart and a stronger body that can handle your problems. In the end, you will welcome challenges and your healthy body and clear mind will help you overcome and solve problems wisely and successfully!

5

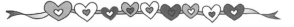

Your Health is Your Wealth – It's Up to You!

Health, like freedom and peace, lasts as long as we exert ourselves to maintain it. It's almost exclusively in your hands whether you enjoy a healthy, vigorous life to a ripe old age or live out a half-alive, non-energetic existence with premature breakdown of health. This poor health condition predominates in civilized countries. Therefore, we find it ironic that so-called civilized nations are said to have a high standard of living. In these countries, coronary (heart) disease is the biggest killer! Apparently their high living standards are not producing health and longevity. See revealing chart page 32. Start The Bragg Healthy Lifestyle today, to ensure a bright, healthy, fulfilled future!

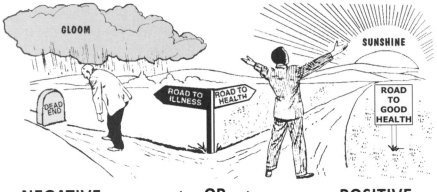

6

NEGATIVE   ⇦ OR ⇨   POSITIVE
The choice of which road to take is up to you.

You alone decide whether to reach a dead end or live a healthy lifestyle for a long, healthy, happy, active life. – Paul C. Bragg

Habits can be right or wrong, good or bad, healthy or unhealthy, rewarding or unrewarding, powerful for good, or powerful for bad. The right or wrong habits and lifestyle decisions, actions, words and deeds are all up to you. Wisely choose your habits and lifestyle, as they can make or break you!
– Patricia Bragg, Pioneer Healthy Lifestyle Educator

To preserve health is a moral and religious duty, for health is the basis for all social virtues. We can't be as useful when not well.
– Dr. Samuel Johnson, Father of Dictionaries, 1709-1784

Healthy Mind Habit: Wake up and say, "Today I am going to be happier, healthier and wiser in my daily living! I am the captain of my life and am going to steer it to living a 100% healthy lifestyle!" Fact is happy people look younger and have fewer health problems! – Patricia Bragg, Pioneer Health Crusader

Chapter 2

One Heart – One Life
To Protect and Treasure

Most people are blessed with a powerful heart at birth. Of course there are always exceptions, like my father, who was born with a weak heart. He needed to fight hard just to survive. But he did survive, persevering to develop a *powerful heart* for a long, active, healthy life!

Your marvelous heart, the perpetual pump that Mother Nature gives us, can go on beating almost indefinitely. Today, right here in the United States there are almost 100,000 people and the count is growing who are 100 years or older. In our research on longevity we have met many people who were 100 to 115 and still living healthy lives. This shows it is possible to enjoy living a long life! What greater treasure and enjoyment is there than a long, happy, healthy, active useful life, and being kind and loving?

Truly it doesn't really matter what your calendar age happens to be. In fact, it might be better all around to forget chronological age and consider only anatomical or physiological age. *We do!* Longevity is really a vascular question. *A man is only as old as his arteries.* Sir William Osler, the Canadian medical teacher and writer, pointed out long ago, *"A man of twenty-eight may have the arteries of a sixty-year-old, and a man of forty may have vessels as degenerated as they could be at eighty."* Remember your arteries are your river of life! Sir Osler stressed the word *degenerated!* Webster's defines degeneration as: *Deterioration of a tissue or an organ in which its vitality is diminished; a process by which normal tissue becomes converted into or replaced by tissue of inferior quality, whether by chemical change of the tissue (true degeneration) or the deposit of abnormal matter in the tissue (infiltration).*

Every day the average heart beats 100,000 times and pumps about 1,800 gallons of blood for nourishing your body. In 70 years this adds up to about 3 billion (faithful) heartbeats. Please be good to your heart and start this Bragg Healthy Heart Program for living a long, happy, healthy fulfilled life!
– Patricia Bragg, Health Crusader & Healthy Lifestyle Educator

Our Miracle Heart and Circulatory System

At birth we are given a heart with clean arteries. It is our unhealthy foods and living habits that cause degeneration. The care we take of our heart can determine the number of years we are going to stay on this earth. It is up to each of us to take special care of our heart so we can make this life a long, healthy and happy one. Health and happiness go hand in hand.

To understand the causes of heart trouble, we must know something about the heart and the circulatory system. The primary function of this cardiovascular system (heart and blood vessels) is to distribute blood through the entire body, carrying a steady flow of nourishment and oxygen to billions of body cells. Just as important, it is responsible to remove toxic wastes from those body cells.

The blood faithfully makes its continual rounds throughout the adult body's 100,000 miles of blood vessels. These vessels connect to all body cells, from the heart itself, to the scalp, down to finger tips and toes. The average person has between *5 and 6 quarts of blood* continually circulating throughout this network. For heart facts see Nova web: *pbs.org/wgbh/nova/body/map-human-heart.html*

Important Heart Parts

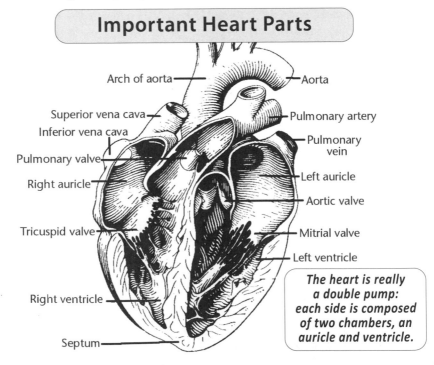

Arch of aorta

Aorta

Superior vena cava

Inferior vena cava

Pulmonary artery

Pulmonary vein

Pulmonary valve

Right auricle

Left auricle

Aortic valve

Tricuspid valve

Mitrial valve

Left ventricle

Right ventricle

Septum

The heart is really a double pump: each side is composed of two chambers, an auricle and ventricle.

Our Miracle Heart is a Powerful Muscle

The heart is a large muscular organ and a very powerful, hard-working miracle! It has to be! *The heart is a muscular (double) pump* whose vital task is to pump the blood and keep it circulating in a life-long journey throughout the body. It's readily apparent that the heart has to be powerful and efficient to do all the endless work required in it's lifetime.

Consider what the heart must do: during rest the blood makes one round trip (through the circulatory system) per minute; during activity or heavy exercise it may make as many as 9 trips a minute in order to supply needed fuel for increased energy and to remove the burnt-out wastes. Even during rest the heart pumps an average of 1,800 gallons of blood every 24 hours, yet it is no bigger than your fist.

The tissues of the body – including the heart – need oxygen to spark the chemical reaction which provides energy, just as a fire needs oxygen before it will burn and generate heat. The blood's important function is to carry oxygenated blood to nourish all the body's tissues.

The oxygen is first picked up in both lungs, then this oxygen-enriched blood (reddish in color) travels to the heart, from there it is then pumped to the tissues where the oxygen content is exchanged for waste. This blood, depleted of oxygen, turns bluish in color as it makes a return trip to the heart to be pumped back into the lungs.

Thus the heart is receiving 2 types of blood simultaneously:

• supplies of **oxygen-enriched blood** from the lungs and
• **oxygen-depleted blood** from the tissues. To keep these two streams separated, the heart chamber is divided in half by a muscular partition called the *septum*. The left and right chambers formed by the septum are each divided into two compartments. The auricle, which has a thin wall, has little pumping action and serves mainly as a reservoir. The other is the ventricle which has a thick, muscular wall and does the main pumping.

The miracle heart pumps approximately 1 million barrels of blood and beats about 3 billion times during a 70 year lifetime – that's enough blood to fill more than 3 super tankers. – Nova Dateline

9

Your Hard-Working Blood Network

The object of the blood circulating is to ensure that all the body's cells will be regularly supplied with food and oxygen, and regularly cleared of toxic substances. To achieve this objective, your 100,000 mile intricate network of blood vessels run throughout your body.

Three varieties of blood vessels are: Arteries, Veins and Capillaries. During blood circulation, Arteries carry blood away from heart. Capillaries connect arteries to veins. Veins finally carry blood back to the heart. All vary greatly in size, just as do streams and creeks that flow into larger rivers.

The largest blood vessel is the *aorta,* the artery which acts as the main supply pipe leading directly out of the heart and from which – through numerous branches – all parts of the body are eventually supplied with blood. The smallest tubes of both the arteries and the veins are called *capillaries* – they're so tiny that most are only visible under a microscope. Through the body's 10 billion capillaries the last of the food and oxygen is exchanged and the return transfer is made into the veins. The veins then carry the oxygen-depleted blood and toxic wastes back to the heart for purification. On the way to the heart, most of the wastes are deposited in the kidneys for elimination from the body through the urine. Carbon dioxide, another impurity, is expelled through the lungs.

Blood Purification for Life-Giving Oxygen

When the blood – which is now full of impurities collected from the tissues of the body – returns to the heart through the veins, it is pumped out at once through a large artery into the lungs. There the blood sheds the carbon dioxide and absorbs the life-giving oxygen the lungs inhaled. (Don't poison this air with tobacco smoke! Read the Bragg *Super Power Breathing* Book.) The newly oxygenated blood then returns to the heart to be pumped out through the aorta to the body.

Heart rate is high in newborns and declines with age. Heart rate can increase among senior citizens. Females generally have slightly higher heart rates than males. Physical activity can lower your resting heart rate, which is important because a slower beating heart is more energy efficient than one that beats rapidly.

Blood circulation is not simple. It follows a design which resembles a figure 8. *There are actually two entirely separate circulations, both go away from and back to the heart.* The *greater* circulatory cycle goes to tissues, limbs, internal organs, and back to the heart. The *lesser* one goes only through the lungs and then back to the heart. Pressure in the blood vessels is naturally much greater in the arteries than in the veins, because the arteries channel the blood pumped out of the heart.

A Healthy Heart Has Steady, Rhythmic Beats

The lower part of your heart is slightly to the left side of your upper body, so it's easier to hear the heartbeat by listening on the left side of the chest. The heartbeat actually originates in the middle of the neck region and descends from the mid-line into the chest. The heart is in the center of the chest. Myths about sleeping on your left side for fear of compressing the heart are nonsense. The best position for sleeping is on your back! (See page 173.)

A healthy heartbeat keeps a steady pumping rhythm, called the *pulse.* The pulse rate is usually measured at the wrist, where one of the main arteries lies near the surface. *The normal adult pulse rate is from 60-72 beats per minute.* Between each heart beat there is $1/6$ of a second rest, thus when a person has lived for 50 years, their wise heart (pump) has rested 8 of those years!

11

The Heart Has It's Own Intelligent Brain

We often hear the phrase, *I know in my heart it's true.* This indicates that we know that our heart is more than just a pump. It can beat on its own without connection to the brain. It starts to form in the fetus before there is a brain! Scientists don't know what triggers the self-initiated heartbeat. Revolutionary heart research is emerging. The Institute of HeartMath in Boulder Creek, California, **found the heart has its own brain and nervous system.** In the 1970's, Fels Research Study found that the *brain in the*

A low resting pulse rate of about 55 beats per minute or lower rather than 70 beats or higher, indicates that your heart can pump more efficiently.

Let us be grateful to our family and people who make us happy; they are the charming gardeners who make our souls blossom. – Marcel Proust

head was obeying messages from the *brain in the heart*. The heart carries intricate messages that affect our emotions, physical health and quality of life! Our heart has the capacity to *think for itself*. The brain's ability to process information and make decisions is affected by how we emotionally react to a situation. See web: *HeartMath.org*.

These dedicated researchers discovered a critical link between the heart and emotions. When the heart responds to emotions such as anger, frustration or anxiety, heart rhythms become incoherent and more jagged; blood vessels constrict, blood pressure rises and the immune system is weakened. Researchers found that many heart failures were precipitated by gross emotional upsets. However, when we feel positive emotions such as love and caring, the heart rhythms become coherent and smoother; thus, enhancing healthy communication between the heart and the brain. Positive heart rhythms produce beneficial effects to cardiovascular efficiency, enhanced immunity, nervous system and hormonal balance. As we learn to become more heart intelligent and improve the emotional balance and heart/brain coherence in ourselves, we will enhance our levels of mental clarity, physical energy and productivity with more daily peace, happiness and a better quality of life!

A key factor in stress is a lack of time. In fact, 75 to 90% of all visits to physicians result from *stress-related* disorders, according to American Institute of Stress. We must utilize our time more wisely, and restore balance in our lives. Researchers found that by *locking in* to positive feelings associated with the heart, such as love, faith, joy, hope, gratitude and appreciation, we can facilitate a more perfect mental, physical, spiritual and emotional balance!

Scientists assumed and most of us were taught that it was only the brain that sent information and issued commands to the heart, but now we know that it works both ways. The heart and head communicate via a number of pathways. Between them they continually exchange critical information that influences how our miracle body functions.

One important way the heart can speak to and influence the brain is when the heart is coherent – generating a stable, sine-wavelike pattern in its rhythms. When your heart is coherent, the body, including the brain, begins to experience all sorts of benefits, among them greater mental clarity and intuitive ability, including better decision-making skills. – See more at: TheHealersJournal.com

Chapter 3

What is a Heart Attack?

The healthy heart is a model of efficiency and perfection. When people don't watch their diet and don't exercise regularly, the walls of their arteries become cluttered with deposits of a wax-like fatty substance called cholesterol. This damages the arteries, forms scar tissue and traps more cholesterol and mineral deposits. This condition is known as *atherosclerosis*. Instead of being as healthy and flexible as they need to be for the pulsing blood flow, the arterial walls become hard and brittle, since the accumulating deposits narrow the channel through which blood must pass. All of this slows down the circulation of blood and may even cause the formation of a clot, which blocks the blood's flow.

Normal Artery Compared to Clogged Artery

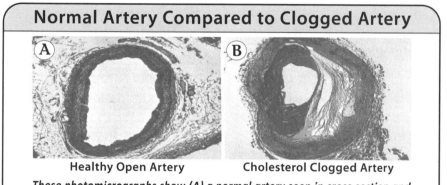

Healthy Open Artery   Cholesterol Clogged Artery

These photomicrographs show (A) a normal artery seen in cross section and (B) a diseased artery in which the channel is partially occluded by atherosclerosis.

13

When a clot forms in one of the heart arteries it creates a serious condition called *coronary thrombosis*, or *coronary occlusion*. The affected part of the heart is deprived of blood circulation. Failing to get nourishment and oxygen, it then ceases to function. This is when a deadly heart attack occurs. *Coronary heart disease* is when potentially deadly cholesterol-rich plaque builds up in arteries, impeding the blood flow.

Thousands of people every year pay thousands of dollars for state-of-the-art testing to learn their risk for heart disease. However, experts say fresh vegetables and fruits and a health club membership are better buys than any lab test. People who eat a diet low in fat and cholesterol and rich in healthy plant foods, who don't smoke, who exercise regularly, and keep their weight and blood pressure in normal range are less likely to have a heart attack than those who don't, despite any genetic tendency toward heart disease. – Harvard Health Letter • Health.Harvard.edu/

Heart Information by Dr. James Balch*

- **Angina Pectoris:** refers to the pain or feeling of a tightness, pressure in the chest. This is a warning sign of an impending heart attack. The pain may be mild or severe.

- **Arrhythmias:** electrical disorders that disrupt the heart's natural rhythm. Palpitations happen when the heart beats out of sequence. The victim feels as if their heart is skipping beats. Studies show magnesium can correct irregular heart beats and save lives of heart patients.

- **Cardiac Arrest:** occurs when the heart stops beating. The blood supply is then stopped to the brain and the victim loses consciousness. Unsuspected coronary artery disease is often the cause of these attacks. Victims will experience brief dizziness followed by unconsciousness.

- **Congestive Heart Failure:** happens when a damaged heart becomes fatigued and is unable to pump effectively. This heart exhaustion results in fluid accumulation in the lungs, labored breathing and swelling in lower legs.

- **Fibrillation:** arterial fibrillation and flutter, heart palpitations or enhanced awareness of heart beating. Dizziness and fainting spells often accompany fibrillation.

- **Myocardial Infarction:** is the medical term for a heart attack. Blood clots causing narrowed coronary artery, cutting off nutrients and oxygen to the heart for a period of time.

- **Ischemic Heart Disease:** is caused by arteriosclerosis, in which fatty deposits along the walls of the arteries obstruct the blood flow to the heart. Sections of the heart muscle may die in those suffering from chronic ischemia. It can lead to angina, myocardial infarction (heart attack), cardiac arrhythmias or congestive heart failure.

- **Ischemic Stroke:** A clot lodges in either the carotid artery or smaller artery branching out from it. A clot buster known as Tissue Plasminogen Activator (TPA) is miraculous. It is used by cardiologists, hospitals and emergency clinics! TPA breaks up clots and dissolves them in 71% of patients when administered within 3 hours of an ischemic stroke! Diagnosing stroke symptoms quickly is crucial for recovery!

---

*Excerpts from "Prescription for Nutritional Healing" – by James Balch, M.D.
"Bragg Health Books were My Conversion to The Healthy Way."

What is a Stroke?

A stroke can originate from the same causes as a heart attack. The arteries become clogged and narrow because of cholesterol and mineral deposits on the arterial walls, hindering free passage of blood. This statement is true and not to be carelessly ignored – *"A man is as old as his arteries."*

Pressure of the blood trying to force its way through the blockage further irritates the artery walls and creates conditions which give rise to blood clots! When a clot breaks off from the artery lining wall into the bloodstream it can slow or completely block blood flow. If a complete blockage occurs in the vital arteries that feeds the heart muscle, the result is a heart attack or ***coronary thrombosis.*** ***Cerebral thrombosis*** (the most common type of stroke) occurs when a blood clot forms and blocks blood flow in an artery supplying blood to part of the brain (sometimes called *a heart attack in the head.*) ***Cerebral hemorrhage***, a stroke which occurs when an artery in the brain bursts, flooding the surrounding tissue with blood. ***Hemorrhagic strokes*** include bleeding within the brain and bleeding between inner and outer layers of the tissue covering the brain. ***Transient Ischemic Attacks*** (or TIAs) greatly diminish blood flow and can last only a couple of minutes. ***Massive Ischemic Strokes*** cause paralysis, difficulty speaking and potentially death. High blood pressure is a major risk factor.

After a stroke occurs the blood supply to part of the brain is reduced or completely cut off. When the nerve cells in that part of the brain are deprived of an oxygenated blood supply, they cannot function and the part of the body controlled by these nerve cells cannot function either. The brain begins to die. Movements can be severely restricted, as well as the ability to speak. The afflicted areas resulting from a stroke depend upon which part of the brain is affected and the seriousness or extent of the damage.

Strokes are a major cause of disability and death among women 50 and older. Strokes can be fatal. It can also produce paralysis of one side or a portion of the body or a single limb. A *lighter* stroke may cause difficulty in moving the arms or legs, in speaking or may result in loss of memory.

High blood pressure is known to be an important risk factor for a stroke.

Thousands Yearly Become Victims of Strokes

Although this disorder is frequently associated with the later years of life, this is not necessarily an affliction of old age. Sadly, this has become an all too common affliction for those in their 30's and 40's. *StrokeDoctor.com/stroke*

Recovery After a Stroke Is Important

After a stroke, the damaged nerve cells may recover or their functions may be taken over by other brain cells. Some victims may suffer serious damage that it will take a dedicated effort to make even a partial recovery. It's important that immediate attention to proper diet and exercise begins! We have seen miracles with stroke victims regaining full use of affected muscles with speech, physical therapy, and massage treatments. Hyperbaric oxygen therapy is also very important and should begin as soon as possible to aid rehabilitation and speed recovery! Prolonged inactivity impairs circulation and makes recovery more difficult! The victim can use his own hands (even if one hand) to massage affected areas 3-6 times daily to bring them back to health. Miracles will happen!

16

How to Recognize Signs of a Stroke

Ask these 3 simple questions: (1) Ask individual to SMILE. (2) Ask person to SPEAK a simple sentence. (3) Ask him or her to RAISE both arms and stick out tongue. If their tongue is "crooked" or goes to one side or the other, that is an indication of a stroke. If they have trouble with ANY of these tasks, call 911 – FAST! and describe these symptoms to dispatcher. If a cardiologist or neurologist can get to a stroke victim within 3 hours they can usually reverse the effects of a stroke!

I've seen partially paralyzed people carried into the hyperbaric oxygen chamber and often walk out after first treatment! – Dr. David Steenblock • StrokeDoctor.com

New research has found that if blood pressure is consistently controlled after an initial stroke, the risk of second stroke can be reduced by more than 50%.

Patients treated with the antibiotic "Minocycline", within 6-24 hours after a stroke, had significantly fewer disabilities, according to a study published in "BMC Neuroscience". Minocycline helps reduce stroke damage by inhibiting white blood cells that can destroy brain tissue & blood vessels. – news-medical.net

What is Angina Pectoris? A Serious Warning!

When one of the heart's arteries is temporarily deprived of blood and oxygen, it goes into a spasm, causing sharp chest pain! Angina chest pain is the most common symptom of heart disease, especially in women. In the Framingham Heart Study (see: *www.FraminghamHeartStudy.org*) women were two times more likely to develop Angina pain as their first symptom of heart disease than a sudden heart attack.* This is your heart's warning pain, crying for a lifestyle change to a healthy diet, fasting, exercise, etc. Usually these spasms last only a few seconds, but sometimes 3-5 minutes, and rarely more than 15-20 minutes. These are serious warnings! Please heed these warning signs listed below!

Warning Signs of Heart Problems

- *Pain or discomfort in your chest, abdomen, back, neck, jaw or arms.* Such symptoms may be signs of an inadequate supply of blood and oxygen to your heart muscle due to potentially serious conditions such as atherosclerotic plaque buildup in your coronary arteries. 17

- *Nausea during or after exercise.* This can result from a variety of causes, but it may signify a cardiac abnormality.

- *Unaccustomed shortness of breath during exercise.* Although this may be related to respiratory problems (asthma, etc.), it could also be a signal of heart trouble.

- *Dizziness or fainting.* This could be a sign of a serious problem – and warrants immediate medical consultation.

- *An irregular pulse.* If you notice what appears to be extra heartbeats or skipped beats, please notify your doctor.

- *A very rapid heart rate at rest.* If your heart rate is 100 beats per minute or higher, report this to your doctor.

*For women the warning signs and symptoms can often be different. For more information see pages 55-58.

ANGINA OCCURS: when the heart muscle "calls for help" because not enough blood is getting to the heart muscle! Angina symptoms usually occur during exercise or stress, when there is a temporary reduction of blood flow to the heart. The symptoms usually resolve with rest. The good news is that angina can be treated with lifestyle changes and medication. A HEART ATTACK OCCURS: when there is a sudden, permanent blockage of the flow of blood to the heart.

Understanding Rheumatic Heart Disease

Rheumatic Heart Disease is a condition in which the heart valves are damaged by rheumatic fever. Rheumatic fever begins with strep throat caused by Group A *Streptococcus* bacteria. Rheumatic fever is an inflammatory disease. It can affect many of the body's connective tissues – especially those of the heart, joints, brain or skin. Anyone can get acute rheumatic fever, but it usually occurs in children 5 to 15 years old. The incidence of rheumatic fever is low in the U.S. and most other developed countries. However, it continues to be a leading cause of cardiovascular death in the developing world.

18

The Kidney's Role in Heart Attacks

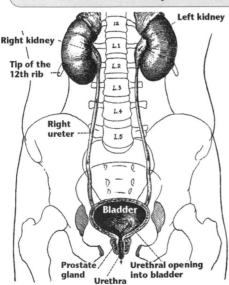

Left kidney
Right kidney
Tip of the 12th rib
12
L.1
L.2
L.3
L.4
L.5
Right ureter
Bladder
Prostate gland
Urethra
Urethral opening into bladder

When the circulation of blood into the kidneys is impeded, their function is seriously impaired. They are soon unable to efficiently eliminate the built-up toxins that accumulate in the blood. The body's vital fluid balance then gets upset and sick. This overburdens the arteries and leads to their breakdown. Millions depend on dialysis. Vitamin C and Chelation Therapy helps (see pages 188-192).

Be Prepared for Heart Emergencies

Because heart attacks come on suddenly, you should be prepared for such an emergency . . . whether it happens to you or someone near you! *If you have been warned that you are a potential heart attack victim* – it is wise to have a portable oxygen supply, such as *Lif-O-Gen®* with you. It is an investment that may save your life or life of a loved one! It is lightweight (3 lbs.) and easily administered (*lifogen.com*).

Everyone should be prepared to aid a heart attack victim in an emergency by calling 911 and if trained giving immediate emergency treatment until professionals arrive! The Red Cross, Fire Departments and many schools offer CPR and First Aid courses, and other life-saving skills. Such knowledge may help you save lives.

Hands-Only™ CPR Can and is Saving Lives!

Most people who experience cardiac arrest at home, work or in a public location die because they don't receive immediate CPR from someone on the scene. As a bystander, don't be afraid. Learning CPR and First Aid skills can help the chances of surviving cardiac arrest with good brain function and are better when bystanders focus on "Hands-Only™ CPR," a Japanese study affirmed. The Hands-Only™ technique may be more effective than conventional CPR in the early phase of sudden cardiac arrest.

An Automated External Defibrillator (AED) offers a fast miracle for victims of sudden cardiac arrest! Cardiac Arrest survival rates (increase) doubled greatly when a trained bystander is able to quickly use an AED rather than awaiting emergency responders. The FAA has decided most passenger planes will carry an AED. Medical Centers, big business, universities, schools, churches, cruise ships, etc. are advised to have one in their First Aid Kits too. See Heart Smart Devices and Supplies (*HeartSmart.com*).

IN EMERGENCY – 1 tsp Cayenne Powder in water or Cayenne Tincture Drops under tongue may help bring person out of heart attack and 15 drops Hawthorn Extract every 15 minutes. – See web: HealthyHealing.com

EVERY MINUTE COUNTS! When someone has a heart attack, it's important to recognize what's happening. Immediately get expert help. Call 911 the paramedics arrive in moments.

If you witness a person collapse having a heart attack – The American Heart Association recommends you call 911 – FAST. If someone nearby is trained and able to start CPR – they should start assisting immediately. If the heart can be kept going, medications usually help strengthen the heart enough so slowly the body can re-route blood to damaged heart muscle through other tiny vessels! This re-routing miracle process, called collateral circulation, helps keep many heart-attack victims alive.

Heimlich Maneuver Jumpstarts Lungs & Heart

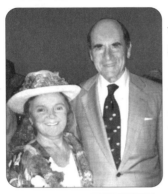

Dr. Henry J. Heimlich with Patricia Bragg in Honolulu

My father and I want to do all we can to ensure that all people are able to get the oxygen they need.

Many of you are familiar with the famous Heimlich Maneuver as a technique for saving choking victims. Since 1974, this procedure has saved *over 100,000* lives just in the United States. This maneuver, developed by Dr. Henry Heimlich, is performed by pressing upward on the diaphragm. This compresses the lungs, causing a flow of air that helps push the choking object out that is blocking the airway. Recent evidence and research has suggested the Heimlich Maneuver is effective in restoring breathing in more emergency situations than just choking. Our friends Dr. Heimlich along with his wife Jane Murray Heimlich *(the daughter of famous Arthur and Katherine Murray who taught America to dance)* dedicated their lives to educating the world about the life-saving Heimlich Maneuver.

Everyone should know the versatile Heimlich Maneuver, for it is life-saving.

Million Hearts® is a national initiative to prevent 1 million heart attacks and strokes by 2022. Million Hearts® brings together communities, health systems, nonprofit organizations, federal agencies, and private-sector partners from across the country to fight heart disease and stroke and to improve care and empower Americans to make heart-healthy choices.
For more info see web: MillionHearts.hhs.gov.

20

Prevention is Far Better than the Cure!

. . . and always more successful! This is why we keep stressing living The Bragg Healthy Lifestyle! You must banish the notion that age alone damages your heart and blood vessels. Remember age is not toxic! It's not a force, but a measure. Live so healthy that you will never suffer a stroke or heart attack! You know what your enemies are – tobacco, excess weight, stimulants such as coffee, tea, alcohol and cola drinks, fatty – unhealthy foods, sugars, table salt, salty foods and lack of ample healthy heart foods and daily exercise!

What Can You Do Today to Reduce Your Vulnerability to a Heart Attack or Stroke?

There are many factors which can lead to stroke or heart attack such as: hypertension, smoking, heavy alcohol or caffeine consumption, overuse of aspirin, medications and drugs, heavy fat, salty, fried-food diet and being overweight.

Thousands of heart attacks and strokes occur every day in the U.S.! You should start immediately to prevent a future heart attack or stroke! The prevention of a heart attack is basically a life-long job of healthy lifestyle living to prevent the slow accumulation of deposits that can clog the arteries. If you are serious about avoiding a heart attack or stroke, you can begin this *Bragg Heart Fitness Program* right now.

Many Cardiologists prescribe aspirin for its anti-clotting factor. We don't! They claim it may reduce heart attacks by 30% by reducing blood clotting. Caution: Aspirin may affect the natural clotting process too much. Some people develop serious stomach problems and gastro-intestinal bleeding. Instead they need immediate lifestyle changes for a healthier heart! Also, taking aspirin does not lower cholesterol or blood pressure!

The first thing you need to work for are clean arteries! The inner lining of a healthy person's arteries are smooth and flexible so blood (your river of life) can flow easily.

To beat the odds of a heart attack – faithfully live The Bragg Healthy Lifestyle that promotes healthy HDL/Cholesterol ratio and Triglyceride levels.

Take Time for 12 Things

1. Take time to **Work** –
   it is the price of success.
2. Take time to **Think** –
   it is the source of power.
3. Take time to **Play** –
   it is the secret of youth.
4. Take time to **Read** –
   it is the foundation of knowledge.
5. Take time to **Worship** –
   it is the highway of reverence and
   washes the dust of earth from our eyes.
6. Take time to **Help and Enjoy Friends** –
   it is the source of happiness.
7. Take time to **Love and Share** –
   it is the one sacrament of life.
8. Take time to **Dream** –
   it hitches the soul to the stars.
9. Take time to **Laugh** –
   it is the singing that helps life's loads.
10. Take time for **Beauty** –
    it is everywhere in nature.
11. Take time for **Health** –
    it is the true wealth and treasure of life.
12. Take time to **Plan** –
    it is the secret of being able to have time
    for the first 11 things.

22

YOUR BIRTHRIGHT
HEALTH
CULTIVATE IT

**Have an
Apple
Healthy Life!**

3 John 2

*Teach me thy way, LORD, lead me in a straight path,
because of my oppressors. – Psalm 27:11*

Chapter 4

Cholesterol & Free Radicals

Importance of Low Blood Cholesterol Levels

Every nation that lives on a modern commercial diet is eating its way into the high cholesterol danger zone of heart attacks. Studies conducted by the greatest medical authorities around the world indicate the shocking dangers of high blood cholesterol levels (see recommended levels inside front cover.) The U.S. has the highest known average blood cholesterol level in the world, and is generally credited with the dubious honor of being the *birthplace of the coronary epidemic!* This is a serious reason for Americans to take action right away!

Americans Love High Cholesterol Foods

Americans love these cholesterol disasters: steaks, big slices of roast beef, thick slices of ham, ribs, pork chops, fried chicken, bacon, and luncheon meats, as well as cheese, ice cream, whipped cream, sour cream, milk, butter, eggs, commercial pies and pastries, candy, french fries, gravies, potato chips and salad dressings made with saturated oils.

All these favorite American foods have a lot of *hard or saturated fats,* primarily of animal origin. These saturated fats are *high in cholesterol.* Consequently, the average blood cholesterol index in the U.S. today is between 230 and 260 – far above the *safety levels.* High cholesterol levels have definitely been established as the *forerunners* of most heart attacks.

Remember the amount of cholesterol in your blood tells you of the risk you are taking of developing a serious coronary ailment or having a heart attack or stroke. It is *the barometer of your life-span.* It's important and wise that adults keep their cholesterol at a safe, normal level (page 24).

Choose a diet low in fat, saturated fat, cholesterol and eat no trans-fats. Trans-fats are found in margarine, vegetable shortening, fried foods, etc. Some dietary fat is needed for good health. Sources of healthy fats include: Olive oil, almonds, pecans, avocados, etc. Healthy fats supply energy, essential fatty acids and promote absorption of fat-soluble vitamins A, D, E and K. Be aware that high levels of saturated fat and cholesterol in diets are linked to increased cholesterol levels and greater risk for heart disease. – Health.gov

Some Blood Cholesterol is Normal

It is perfectly normal to have a certain amount of fat and cholesterol in your bloodstream. Called *lipoproteins,* they are necessary for the upkeep of the body. However, trouble begins when you have an excess of fat clogging your body's pipes. This is why it is essential to master and wisely live The Bragg Healthy Lifestyle; it helps keep your blood cholesterol levels healthy and normal.

Every cell in the body needs some cholesterol to function properly. Cell walls, or membranes, need cholesterol in order to produce hormones, vitamin D, and bile acids that help to digest fat. But the body needs only a limited amount of cholesterol to meet its needs. When too much is present health problems such as heart disease may develop. Cholesterol is not the same as fat. Produced in the liver, cholesterol is delivered through the bloodstream to all the various cells of the body. However, the cells take only what cholesterol they need; any excess remains in the bloodstream. The unused, not needed cholesterol eventually collects in your circulatory system as plaque deposits that clog artery walls.

24

Good news – your liver rarely produces more cholesterol than the body needs! The bad news is that it can enter the body by more ways than the liver's activity. Your lifestyle and what you eat also greatly influences cholesterol levels!

This fatty substance, cholesterol, is found in the liver, brain, nerves, bile and blood of all humans. Eating meat and dairy products (where cholesterol is found) can raise your cholesterol levels. When this is beyond the amount your body needs, the excess remains in the bloodstream and collects along arterial passages. *Warning: this arterial cholesterol buildup may cause serious cardiovascular blockage and even death!*

Recommended Heart Health Tests (for Adults):

- **Total Cholesterol:** 180 mg/dl or less is optimal
- **LDL Cholesterol:** 130 mg/dl or less is optimal • **HDL Cholesterol:** 50 mg/dl or more
- **Triglycerides:** 150 mg/dl or less is normal level
- **HDL/Cholesterol Ratio:** 5.0 or less • **Triglycerides/HDL Ratio:** below 2
- **Homocysteine:** 6-9 micromoles/L
- **CRP (C-Reactive Protein high sensitivity):**
  - • 1 mg/L = low risk • 1-3 mg/L = average risk • over 3 mg/L = high risk
- **Diabetic Risk Tests:**
  - • **Glucose:** (do 12 hour food fast) 80-100 mg/dl • **Hemoglobin A1c:** 6% or less
- **Blood Pressure:** 120/70 mmHg is good for adults

Two Types of Cholesterol – HDL and LDL

Researchers discuss the two main types of cholesterol:

FIRST are *high-density lipoproteins (HDL)*, known as *"good cholesterol."* The lower your total cholesterol level, and the higher your HDL as a proportion of this, the lower your risk of heart attack. The ratio of total cholesterol to HDL should be less than 4 to 1. Researchers believe HDLs travel through the bloodstream collecting *bad cholesterol and disposing of it.*

SECOND are the *low-density lipoproteins (LDL)*, often referred to as *"bad cholesterol."* When LDLs occur in excess, they can dangerously coat and clog arterial walls and dramatically increasing your risk of a heart attack or stroke. LDL cholesterol is also very dangerous in another way – when exposed to heat and oxygen, these cholesterol molecules slowly change. When this occurs in fats, we call this process *going rancid*. When fats go rancid, their LDLs become infested with the *harmful free radicals*.

What Are Harmful Free Radicals?

There is much talk about "free radicals" the toxic oxygen molecules that attack the body's cells. These dangerous sources of free radical contamination substances (page 27) cause many health problems and early ageing! The health risk they pose is so great, Dr. Julian Whitaker says:

Free radicals (toxic oxygen molecules), are a primary cause of heart disease – #1 health problem facing the world today!

What Causes Excessive Free Radicals?

Free radicals can be caused by any number of factors including a poor diet. Fatty and sugary foods and drinks, junk and processed foods are just a few of the causes of free radicals. Smoking, pollution, radiation, herbicides and pesticides also cause excessive free radicals to form. This is why it's so important to only eat organic fruits and veggies.

Sadly, almost 40% of Americans have cholesterol levels over 200.
If cholesterol is over 200: each point it's lowered, heart attack risk is reduced 2%.

Smoking and obesity lower good HDL cholesterol. HDL can be raised with exercise and foods which are rich in vitamin C. – www.pcrm.org

Free Radicals are Cancer Producers

Free radicals are very dangerous elements that can alter and change food molecules. With LDLs (found in all animal proteins and their by-products), free radicals change the original cholesterol structure into more than 400 different harmful, toxic substances! Once in the body, free radicals roam widely, attacking and damaging cells. The free radicals may attack DNA (your genetic inheritance) causing cancer or even birth defects; in the pancreas they can cause diabetes; in the eye they can cause cataracts, and in the blood and blood vessels they can cause cardiovascular disease. Free radicals are introduced into the body through your environment, as well as by your diet. See *Toxic Free Radical Catalysts* list – page 27.

Free Radicals Cause Premature Ageing

Most risk factors for coronary heart disease, such as high blood pressure or smoking, create free radicals that prevent the inner walls of blood vessels from producing nitric oxide. This is necessary for proper blood vessel expansion and contraction. A free radical is an unstable atom, molecule or ion that reacts with other molecules in destructive ways! An excess of free radicals causes premature ageing and other serious medical conditions, depending on which tissues are being attacked.

Free Radical Catalysts Are Dangerous

Don't be a passive victim of destructive free radicals! Take heart, avoid these free radical contaminations. Also avoid the unhealthy foods listed on page 144. Living The Bragg Healthy Lifestyle helps arrest free radicals and ageing, and earns you a healthier heart and body for enjoying a longer, healthier life! Faithfully guard and protect your precious body and your health! The substances on the next page are dangerous sources of free radical contamination. It's healthiest for you to avoid them!

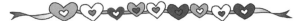

Healthy diets (salads, veggies, etc.) leave less room for foods like sugar pastries, cookies, ice cream and candy which can negatively influence your health, weight, blood cholesterol and thereby raise diabetes and heart disease risks!

Eliminate Exposure to Toxic Free Radicals:

- **Aluminum** – in antacids, deodorants, baking powder, tap water, deodorants, cans, foils, pots, pans, and in many drugs
- **Cadmium** – most common in batteries, but also found in cigarette smoke, coffee, gasoline, and metal pipes
- **Carbon Monoxide** – auto exhaust, cigarette smoke, smog
- **Chlorine** – tap water, swimming pools and table salt
- **Copper** – tap water, toothpastes and dental work
- **Lead** – dyes, gasoline fumes, paint, plumbing, auto exhaust
- **Mercury** – amalgam (silver) fillings, fish, paint, cosmetics
- **Nitrates and Nitrites** – used in many processed foods, meats, etc. as a preservative. Also found in tap water
- **Petroleum Products** – fuels, solvents, polishes and paints
- **Pesticides** – Dioxin, heptachlor, dieldrin, and DDT are in most fruits and veggies. This is why you should go organic!
- **Polynuclear Hydrocarbons** – asphalts, fuels, oils and greases. Also deep-fried, char-broiled and BBQ foods
- **Radiation** – environmental radiation, TV and cell phones
- **Synthetic Drugs** – antibiotics, painkillers, barbiturates
- **Preservatives, Artificial Colorings and Food Additives**
- **Synthetic Materials** – such as polyester, acetate, plastic, etc.

27

Heavy metals in your body multiply those free radical chain reactions several thousand, possibly several million times. When a free radical molecule hits a metal atom in your body, the effect is multiplied many-fold. This is partly why it is so important to remove toxic metals from your body.

THE DANGERS OF FREE RADICALS: They trigger a damaging chain reaction. "Free radicals are dangerous because they don't just damage one molecule," says Blumberg (from WebMD.com). "One free radical can set off a whole chain reaction. When a free radical oxidizes a fatty acid, it changes that fatty acid into a free radical, which then damages another fatty acid. It's a very rapid chain reaction." These external attacks can overwhelm the body's natural free-radical defense system. In time, and with repeated free radical attacks that the body cannot stop, that damage can lead to a host of chronic diseases, including cancer, heart disease, Alzheimer's disease, and Parkinson's disease.

When you eat multiple servings of organic fruits and vegetables, you are compensating for the effects of harmful environmental toxins. – WebMD.com.

Living The Bragg Healthy Lifestyle is your insurance policy for health and longevity!

Oxygen and It's Importance

Keeping this list in mind, it's important to talk about oxygen for a moment. Oxygen is an important part of our lives. It's in the air we breathe, water we drink and food we eat. The problem is there isn't enough of it these days.

How is this important? Oxygen plays a vital role in our breathing and metabolic processes. Nutrient compounds inside our cells are oxidized by enzymes and this oxidation process is our main source of well-being. If there is enough oxygen in the body it's very difficult for degenerative diseases to survive.

But since there is a shortage of oxygen (pollution in our cities, carbon monoxide poisoning, etc.) our bodies have to use other "creative" methods to get oxygen. Stress, fear and anxiety cause shallow breathing or even holding our breath. This causes an increase in free radicals. As long as you are living and breathing, there's no way around this. The best thing you can do is start eating more antioxidant rich foods.

Life-Saving Antioxidants Reduce Free Radicals

There is scientific evidence that reducing damage caused by free radicals reduces the effects of ageing and extends your lifespan! Antioxidants are compounds that neutralize the effect of free radicals to prevent them from harming your body. Both antioxidants and free radicals are naturally produced by your body. You can tip the scales in your favor by increasing vital antioxidants through diet rich in vitamin C, E, barley grass, beta carotene (found in green leafy vegetables, yams, sweet potatoes, carrots, etc.), and flavonoids (found in grapeseed extract, bee pollen, milk thistle, ginkgo, etc.). See the list on the next page. The danger of free radicals is immense, so please maximize your intake of super antioxidants (through healthy nutrition and supplements*) and minimize your exposure to toxic "free radical" catalysts.

*SOD – Super Oxide Dismutase, is an antioxidant that helps neutralize free radicals so they are no longer a danger to the body. Also Vitamin A helps protect mucous membranes from damage, helps improve night vision, makes bones, gums and tooth enamel stronger and many more health benefits.

List of Natural Occurring Antioxidant Foods

Antioxidants can be found in a variety of whole foods including organic fruits and vegetables, legumes and whole grains. When we eat these foods, we benefit from a natural defense system that includes: anthocyanins, flavonoids, lutein, lycopene, catechins, selenium, and coenzyme Q10, and vitamins C and E. See: *DoctorOz.com*.

Berries: are a treasure trove of antioxidants, especially blueberries, cranberries and blackberries. Raspberries, strawberries and acai berries are also high on the list. Many antioxidant-rich foods can be identified by their deep natural colors, such as the dark red of ripe raspberries or deep purple of delicious blueberries and blackberries.

Carrots: Another bright vegetable that's high on the antioxidant list is carrots. Fresh, crisp carrots contain large amounts of beta carotene, which is a notable component of many healthy whole foods. Beta carotene helps increase disease-fighting powers of antioxidants and can be found in several fresh fruits as well.

Green Vegetables: All food colors contain some amount of antioxidants, but many green vegetables are especially loaded with antioxidants. Kale, brussels sprouts, spinach, artichokes, asparagus, broccoli and watercress are all strong sources of antioxidants.

29

Kiwi Fruit is Great for Your Heart

Research found that eating just 2-3 kiwi fruits a day may significantly reduce risk of heart disease. The study showed eating kiwi fruit greatly increased blood levels of vitamin C, E and HDL ("good") cholesterol, while lowering the LDL ("bad") cholesterol. Plus, kiwi fruit can lower triglyceride levels by 15%. With its high concentration of antioxidants, it helps prevent cell damage that has been linked to cardiovascular disease, cancer and dementia. In fact, your body actually absorbs antioxidants more effectively from kiwi fruit than from any other antioxidant-rich fruits.

Eating organic green leafy vegetables helps protect against heart attacks. Dark-green leafy veggies such as chard, kale and spinach, yellow vegetables like carrots and squash and yellow fruits like cantaloupe and mango are filled with carotenoids, which is one kind of antioxidant. Citrus fruits, including oranges, lemons and grapefruits contain vitamin C, another antioxidant. Nuts, whole grains, oils from olives, soybean, sunflower and corn contain vitamin E, yet another antioxidant. Be sure to eat ample fresh, organic fruits and veggies!

Grains: though not as high in antioxidants as fresh fruits or vegetables, whole grains are also a valuable source of immunity-boosting compounds. To get the biggest benefit, make sure you choose products that contain 100% whole grains as a first ingredient rather than refined or processed grains. Other whole grains, such as barley, millet, oats and corn, are good sources of antioxidants.

Legumes: many foods that are naturally rich in vitamin E are also rich in antioxidants. Legumes and beans including lentils, soybeans, split peas, and pinto beans contain beneficial amounts of both compounds.

Green Tea: one serving of green tea (decaffeinated) has more antioxidants than a serving of broccoli and also contains substances that neutralize harmful free radicals in the body.

Types of Miracle Working Antioxidants

There are 3 primary types of antioxidants found in nature. These include *phytochemicals* (chart page 140), *vitamins* and *enzymes*. The most powerful antioxidants are found in plants. This is due to fact that plants in *Mother Earth* are exposed to *Father Sun* throughout the day.

Phytochemicals: naturally used by plants to protect themselves against free radicals. Studies show humans who eat sources of phytochemicals also benefit from antioxidant properties of the plant (see pages 139-141).

Vitamin A: is particularly important for improving the immune system, tissue repair, and cholesterol levels.

Vitamin C: Stops free radical chain reaction before it starts; it captures the free radical and neutralizes it.

Vitamin E: is a chain-breaking antioxidant. Wherever it is sitting in a membrane, it breaks the chain reaction.

Beta-carotene: is especially excellent at scavenging free radicals in low oxygen concentration.

Antioxidant Enzymes: superoxide dismutase (SOD), catalase (CAT) and glutathione peroxidase (GPx) serve as your primary line of defense in destroying free radicals.

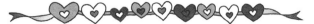

For more info visit web: www.Ageless.co.za/antioxidants.htm

Atherosclerosis – A Fat Hardening Disease

The clogging of the arterial system by excess cholesterol – the deposits of heavy, waxy fat on the artery walls – is called *atherosclerosis*. The components of the word, *atherosclerosis*, are of Greek origin. *Athere* means porridge or mush and refers to the soft fatty material in the core of the plaque; *skelros* means hard and refers to the hard scar-like tissue formation involved in the development of a plaque, and *osis* is a Greek suffix meaning a diseased condition. Therefore, it is a fat hardening disease!

The term *arteriosclerosis* is a group of diseases that cause thickening, blocking and loss of elasticity of the artery wall! Both atherosclerosis and arteriosclerosis are often used interchangeably. Atherosclerosis mostly affects the aorta – the largest blood vessel in the body, and the coronary arteries and the cerebral arteries which supply the brain, legs and abdomen. Atherosclerosis can start with high blood pressure, smoking and increased concentration of fats in the bloodstream.

Rich American Diet is a Killer

Atherosclerosis is not caused by old age, but by diet! Autopsies of American soldiers killed in battle in the Korean and Vietnam Wars revealed the shocking fact that 77% of these soldiers (average ages 18-22) already had atherosclerosis! In contrast, the Koreans and other Asians who died on the same battlefield, under the same conditions, had only an 11% incidence of this disease. It is well known, the traditional Asian diet consists mainly of rice and vegetables and is low in meat and saturated fats.

Saturated fats make up 40% of the caloric intake of the average American diet. Most of these are the commercial, hydrogenated fats – the most clogging, deadly of all fats and are not natural in any sense of the word. It's such a solid fat that it cannot be broken down by the body's 98.6°F heat.

The best natural, unsaturated fats break down at body temperature and don't cause clogging problems. These are perishable foods and don't have a long shelf life. In time, unsaturated fats (oils, etc.) can take on oxygen and become rancid, which gives off a strong odor and bitter taste.

<table>
<thead>
<tr><th rowspan="2">Country</th><th>Women Death Rate
Per 100,000</th><th>% Fat in Relation
to Total Calories</th></tr>
</thead>
<tbody>
<tr><td colspan="3" align="center">

World Death Rates Due to Heart Diseases from Fat in Diet

</td></tr>
</tbody>
</table>

World Death Rates Due to Heart Diseases from Fat in Diet

Country	Women Death Rate Per 100,000	% Fat in Relation to Total Calories
New Zealand	389	39.8
Sweden	235	39.4
Finland	314	39.2
United Kingdom	354	38.4
Denmark	306	38.3
Canada	229	38.0
Norway	266	38.0
Australia	250	37.9
Germany	299	35.6
Belgium	225	35.0
Switzerland	167	33.6
Austria	311	31.3
United States	323	31.1
France	131	29.5 *
Portugal	312	24.5 *
Italy	213	22.3 *
Japan	161	7.9 *

*This chart illustrates the striking difference between New Zealand, U.S. and Japan, the death rate varying by more than 250%. *The lowest four countries use less saturated fats. – From American Heart Association*

32

Beware of Saturated, Hydrogenated Fats!

Hydrogenated, saturated fat remains *stable* because it's impervious to oxygen. In reality, it is embalmed fat! The American consumer has been brainwashed by the large manufacturers into believing they are safe and permanently fresh and healthy! A container of this processed fat will keep for years, because it's impossible for it to turn rancid. Clever ads say these saturated, hydrogenated, processed (erroneously called vegetable) shortenings will not smoke. They also make other clever sales claims which have no relation whatsoever to good nutrition. The same applies to unhealthy margarine made to imitate butter. Some vegetable oils are high in saturated fats, also some tropical oils: palm oil and coconut oil. All hydrogenated oils are high in saturated fat. We use organic extra-virgin olive oil.

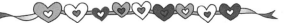

The health and destiny of countries depends on how they eat. – Brillat-Savarin

Animal products also contain substantial amounts of saturated fat, which can cause the liver to produce more cholesterol. Unsaturated fats do not have this effect. Saturated fats are easy to spot – they are solid at room temperature, whereas unsaturated fats are liquid. So, instead of natural, unsaturated fats that will aid health, Americans consume deadly hydrogenated saturated fats, high in cholesterol that coat and clog the bloodstream, especially the arteries. This clogging eventually can cause fatal or crippling clots (thrombosis) in the bloodstream, causing strokes and heart attacks!

Play it Safe – Know Your Cholesterol Levels

There are many simple home cholesterol tests available. These FDA approved tests are over 97% accurate and require only a finger prick.

When you have a complete cholesterol panel ask your doctor for a copy of your HDL, LDL and triglyceride levels (page 24 and inside front cover). These readings determine your main risk factors for heart disease. HDL *good* cholesterol helps protect you from a heart attack. You can help raise your *good* HDL by eating healthy foods, exercising, losing any excess weight and not smoking. An HDL less than 35 mg-dl puts you at a health risk. The LDL or *bad* cholesterol should not exceed 130 mg-dl. To lower undesirable LDL levels, seek a low-fat, low-cholesterol, low-saturated fat diet. Triglyceride levels over 200 mg-dl, are dangerous and associated with obesity, sweets, fats and alcohol intake.

33

The American Heart Association recommends the following guidelines to a healthier heart:

- Consume less than 300 mg of cholesterol per day.
- Consume 30% or fewer calories from fat.
- Consume 10 or less calories from saturated fat.

Saturated fats are the hard fats found mostly in animal products such as lard, butter and fatty meat, as well as in vegetable oils such as coconut and palm.

People who regularly eat barley see significant reductions in LDL (bad) cholesterol, triglycerides and total cholesterol. – Tufts Health & Nutrition Letter

---

The USA leads the world in heart disease, strokes, cancer and diabetes!

If you want to keep your daily cholesterol count, purchase a fat gram counter and it will help count your cholesterol, total fat and saturated fat. We personally don't count calories, fat grams, etc. We live The Bragg Healthy Lifestyle and it keeps us healthy!

Follow these "Golden Rules" for maintaining safe cholesterol levels: eat only healthy, natural foods; get plenty of exercise; breathe deeply; drink 8 glasses pure distilled water daily; get 8 hours of sleep nightly; fast regularly; and have a positive, happy, mental attitude. Those of you who are at risk of cardiovascular problems – please be aware of your current blood cholesterol levels.

CHOLESTEROL COUNT OF COMMON FOODS

FOOD FROM ANIMAL		FOOD FROM PLANT	
Cholesterol Count	*(mg)*	*Cholesterol Count*	*(mg)*
Beef Liver, 3 oz	410	All beans	0
Eggs, 1 whole	213	All fruits	0
Duck, roasted, 3 oz	197	All grains	0
Chicken Liver, 3 oz	126	All legumes	0
Turkey, roasted, 1 cup	106	All nuts	0
Cheeseburger, 4 oz	104	All seeds	0
Ice Cream, 1 cup	88	All vegetables	0
Pork chop, broil, 3 oz	84	All vegetable oils	0
Beef Steak, 3 oz	77	**Sources:**	
Lamb, roasted, 3 oz	77	**1. Healthy Eating Club**	
Chicken Breast, 3 oz	73	**HealthyEatingClub.org**	
Milk, whole, 1 cup	33	**2. UCSF Medical Center:** ucsfHealth.org/	
Butter, 1 Tblsp	31	education/cholesterol_content_of_foods/	
Cream Cheese, 1 oz	31		

10 Foods That Help Lower Your Cholesterol

If your diet gave you high cholesterol, it can lower it too. Here is a list of foods that can help lower your cholesterol:

- *Oats*. An easy first step to improving your cholesterol.
- *Barley & other whole grains*. Deliver soluble fiber.
- *Beans*. Especially rich in soluble fiber, very versatile food.
- *Eggplant & Okra*. Low-calorie vegetables, good soluble fiber.
- *Nuts*. Eating 2 oz. of raw nuts daily can lower LDL by 5%.
- *Vegetable Oils*. In place of butter or lard helps lower LDL.
- *Apples, grapes, strawberries, citrus*. Pectin-rich lower LDL.
- *Fatty fish*. 2-3 x weekly, deliver LDL lowering omega-3 fats.
- *Fiber supplements*. Psyllium provides 4 grams soluble fiber.

34

Cholesterol is only found in animal products. Fruits, veggies, grains and all other plant foods do not have any cholesterol! – UCSF Medical Center

How Much Cholesterol is in Your Blood?

Too many people today eat a diet overloaded with high cholesterol content of saturated animal fats. When these people increase the burden on their bodies by not exercising enough to burn up even the normal – much less the excess – amount of cholesterol as fuel, their bloodstreams become *choked*. Most people know little about their cholesterol levels. They merrily go on using large quantities of butter on their bread, toast, potatoes and vegetables. They drink great quantities of milk, gobble gallons of ice cream and eat meat, fish, poultry, eggs, chips, french fries, doughnuts, bacon, ham and sausage – *that fill their bloodstreams with excess fat!* Little do they realize their high cholesterol levels can lead them to disaster, and they may be literally eating themselves to death! Millions consume as many as 5 cups of saturated fats daily. Then they wonder why they end up with a heart attack, stroke or other forms of heart trouble – it's clogged arteries!

It has been clinically established that the amount of cholesterol deposited on the walls of the arteries has a direct relationship to the amount of cholesterol in the bloodstream. Thus you can see how clogged the arteries must be when cholesterol levels rise to 270, 320, 380 and higher! Yet these excessive levels are not uncommon today.

Cholesterol and Your Lifespan

One thing that will unquestionably shorten the lifespan is a body that is overburdened with blood fat, an excess of cholesterol! To reiterate: some cholesterol is important to our body processes. The body even manufactures it as extra fuel in emergencies. *Chole* means bile and *sterol* means fatty. Much of the fat we eat is broken down by the liver into cholesterol and excreted into the bile, later to be re-absorbed into the bloodstream for distribution to our tissues.

Experts state "120-180" cholesterol level best: Top medical scientists agree that one's cholesterol level should not be over 180. Some professional opinions . . .
Dr. W.D. Wright of University Nebraska College of Medicine – "150 to 180"
Dr. A.G. Shaper of Makerer College Medical School, Uganda – "170" best
Dr. Bernard Amsterdam, New York State Journal of Medicine – "180 maximum"
Dr. Louis H. Nahum, Yale School of Medicine – "150" & Dr. William Dock, Professor of Medicine at State University New York, – "120-180" is optimal normal range.

Fasting – Quickest Way to Lower Cholesterol

In our opinion, fasting is the quickest and easiest method of lowering cholesterol level. We check our blood cholesterol twice a year. If it tops 180, we fast from 3-7 days and it soon drops below 150. Fasting (see pages 163-170) is an easy way to give the heart and cardiovascular pipes a good cleansing. That's why faithfully each week we fast for a 24-hour period on 5-7 glasses distilled (purified) water and also three vinegar drinks (recipe page 150). For more details on the Science of Fasting, read our book *The Miracle of Fasting*. See book list on back pages for ordering.

Other Ways to Lower Your Cholesterol

Go Vegan: The best way to keep saturated fat intake low and to avoid cholesterol completely is to base your diet mainly on plant foods – grains, beans, vegetables and fruits. A vegan diet is free of all animal products – this means no red meat, poultry, fish, eggs, milk, cheese, yogurt, ice cream, butter, etc. – this yields the lowest risk of heart disease.

Fiber: Soluble fiber helps to slow absorption of some food components such as cholesterol. It also acts to reduce the amount of cholesterol the liver makes. Oats, barley, beans, and some fruits and vegetables are all good sources of soluble fiber. There is no fiber in any animal product.

Maintain Your Ideal Weight: Carrying excess weight can affect one's risk for heart disease! Losing weight helps increase HDL levels (the "good cholesterol"). People who have a large waistline are at a higher risk than those who carry excess weight around the hips and buttocks.

Blood Pressure is also a risk factor for heart disease and can lead to strokes and other serious health problems (see next chapter). Luckily, this is another area where we can take control by watching the foods we eat. A low-fat, high-fiber vegetarian diet can help lower blood pressure.

Smoking: People who smoke have a much higher risk of heart disease than non-smokers. Moderation is not good enough – it is essential to quit smoking! (see pages 84-88).

Exercise: Regular light exercise such as a daily half-hour nature brisk walk, can cut death rates dramatically.

Less Stress: Getting enough rest and learning techniques for stress reduction: meditation, yoga or walking is helpful.

36

Chapter 5

The Dangers of High Blood Pressure & Metabolic Syndrome

The Silent Killer – High Blood Pressure

Each time the heart beats, it exerts a pressure on the veins and arteries called "Blood Pressure." What happens when you blow too much air into a balloon? If it doesn't pop, the overextended balloon becomes thin and delicate. Properly inflated, the balloon can be safely bounced and moved around. A balloon with too much air becomes a pop waiting to happen. Don't let this happen to your vessels and heart.

We need blood pressure for blood to circulate! Too much pressure makes the heart and blood vessels thin and delicate. Increased pressure on arterial walls makes them more susceptible to fatty deposits, and possible stroke or heart attack.

High Blood Pressure is Often Symptomless

37

The dangers of untreated *hypertension* (high blood pressure) can be deadly! If left untreated, the arteries can become hardened, scarred, and less elastic, unable to carry adequate blood to the organs. The heart, brain and kidneys are most vulnerable. High blood pressure is the highest risk factor for stroke and heart disease. High blood pressure causes the heart to enlarge and become less efficient, known as *left ventricular hypertrophy*. Left ventricular hypertrophy is more common in people who have uncontrolled high blood pressure or other heart problems. This dangerous condition can lead to heart attacks. Many connect stress with high blood pressure. Some studies have suggested chronic stress can lead to permanent increases in blood pressure and heart rate (air traffic controllers who have high-pressure jobs, have a 2-4 times higher rate of hypertension and heart problems).

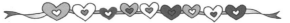

The large network of veins and arteries through which blood circulates needs to be open, clear and strong to keep your blood circulating. High blood pressure is a sign of straining, having to squeeze extra hard to push blood through. This wears you out and your heart, too. Change to The Bragg Healthy Lifestyle.

For a healthy, fit heart, it's wise to keep your blood pressure within the normal 120/70 range. You can manage this with simple dietary and lifestyle changes. Exercise, deep breathing, ample sleep and a healthy diet will help keep your blood pressure under healthy control.

Don't add salt to foods, and avoid prepared foods with high salt, sugar and trans-fat contents. Especially avoid all refined sugars and fat (donuts, cakes, cookies, pies, muffins, etc.)! Never use highly saturated fats. Avoid the fast, nutritionally empty foods so common in our *rush and go* culture. *Eat heart healthy nutritious, longevity foods!*

What Blood Pressure Measurements Mean

There are two types of blood pressure readings. *Systolic* pressure (first figure in reading) refers to pressure exerted by the blood while the heart is pumping; this reading indicates blood pressure at its highest. *Diastolic* pressure (second figure) reads the blood pressure when the heart is at rest in between beats, when the blood pressure is at its lowest. Both readings are important; neither should be high. A normal pressure reads 120 over 70 to 80 (120/70-80), with the systolic pressure measuring 120 mmHg and the diastolic pressure measuring 70 to 80 mmHg.

What Can Happen if . . .
High Blood Pressure is Not Treated?

Untreated high blood pressure can result in:

- Stroke (see page 15)
- Heart failure, an enlarged heart or heart attack
- Kidney disease (see page 18)
- Hemorrhages (bleeding) in the eye blood vessels
- Peripheral vascular disease: the lack of blood circulation in the legs, cramp-like pain in the calves (claudication), or an aneurysm (abnormal enlargement or bulging of an artery caused by damage to or weakness in the blood vessel wall).

If you are not already 1 in 3 of U.S. adults with high blood pressure, the odds are that without intervention, you will be, at some point in your life. In fact, the risk of becoming hypertensive is greater than 90% for individuals in developed countries, according to an editorial in the "Lancet."

Other Possible Dangers of High Blood Pressure

High blood pressure can also affect other areas of the body, leading to such problems as:

• **Bone Loss.** High blood pressure can increase the amount of calcium that's in your urine – this excessive elimination of calcium may lead to loss of bone density (osteoporosis), which in turn can lead to broken bones! The risk is especially increased in older women (page 225).

• **Trouble Sleeping.** Obstructive sleep apnea – a condition in which your throat muscles relax causing you to snore, occurs in more than half of those with high blood pressure (see pages 171-176 on sleep). It's now thought that high blood pressure itself may help trigger sleep apnea. Also, sleep deprivation resulting from sleep apnea can raise your blood pressure. (See bottom of page 175.)

Lowering Blood Pressure Reduces Heart Risk

The International Society of Hypertension unveiled results of the largest hypertension study ever completed, the Hypertension Optimal Treatment (HOT) study. They found lowering one's diastolic blood pressure level to 90 mmHg, can help reduce major cardiovascular risk! Study also found that patients with diabetes, who lowered their diastolic blood pressure level to 80 mmHg, lowered their risk of heart problems! This study amassed 18,790 patients in 26 countries over a 5-year period. According to Dr. Claude Lenfant, director of The National Heart, Lung & Blood Institute, *"Lowering blood pressure beyond traditional levels of 90 mmHg, there's reason to believe that cardiovascular morbidity and mortality can be diminished."* The Study found patients with coronary artery disease, had a 43% reduction in strokes when their blood pressure level was 80 mmHg and lower. High blood pressure is the most common heart disorder and the leading cause of death in America. Over 647,000 deaths per year in persons aged 65-84, are due to cardiovascular disease and more than $219 billion dollars are spent for their terminal medical care and fighting for their life!

Fluctuations in blood pressure may be associated with greater cardiovascular risk.

High Blood Pressure Linked to Mental Decline

High blood pressure can lead to declines in some mental abilities, according to researchers at University of Maine. High blood pressure leads to scarring in blood vessels that has been linked to development of Alzheimer's disease and other dementias. Elevated blood pressure is a strong predictor of changes in brain structure and related cognitive functioning. The researchers examined blood pressure and mental function in 140 men and women ages 40-70. They found that higher levels of blood pressure were associated with greater declines in intelligence tests, visual-spatial abilities and speed of performance!

High Blood Pressure in Adolescence

New Millennium Studies presented at the Scientific Session of The American College of Cardiology found children who are overweight at ages 6 or 7, are more likely to have high blood pressure by adolescence! Researchers studied 200 children for 10 years, examining blood pressure, obesity and metabolic abnormalities. The results showed body mass index (being overweight) correlated strongly to higher blood pressure in children, even after they reached young adulthood. The finding strongly suggests primary overweight prevention may need to begin even before the first day of school, promoting good nutrition, as well as exercise and fitness!

40

How Is High Blood Pressure Treated?

If you have high blood pressure, the goal is to lower blood pressure to less than 140/90 (less than 130/80 for those who have diabetes or kidney disease). To do this:

- **Eat healthy foods** such as fruits and veggies (pg. 136)
- **Lose weight**, if you are overweight (see pages 64-68)
- **Limit alcohol** to no more than one drink each day
- **Exercise regularly** (see pages 89-98)
- **Quit smoking** (see pages 84-88)
- **Have blood pressure checked** regularly

Study found that young adults (18-30) with healthy blood pressure go on to have better thinking and memory skills in midlife than their peers with higher blood pressure. Higher blood pressure readings early in life were associated with poor performance on memory, learning and decision processing speed.

High Blood Pressure Drugs Pose Health Risks

When it comes to dealing with high blood pressure, most Western doctors turn first to drug treatments. They rely mainly on pharmaceuticals – *diuretics* and *beta-blockers*. Drug *diuretics* (with side effects – see below) lower blood pressure by reducing the volume of blood. With less blood, the pressure in the arteries decreases. The other commonly prescribed type of drug, *beta blocker* (also with side effects – see below) works on the autonomic nervous system. Beta blockers slow heart rate, which reduces the pressure by reducing the amount of blood the heart pumps.

Diuretics & Beta Blockers Have Side Effects

These drugs both claim to be helpful remedies for high blood pressure, but don't be too sure. **Diuretics** relieve one problem only to cause several others: They deplete blood of certain essential minerals, increase blood's cholesterol level, and increase blood's thickness, stickiness and acidity. These factors increase heart attack risk. Studies show that death rates increase with heavy diuretic use.

41

What about **beta blockers**? Though their cardiovascular side-effects are less pronounced than diuretics, beta blockers are known for causing impotence, depression and fatigue. Beta blockers can also affect your cholesterol and triglyceride levels, causing a slight increase in triglycerides and a modest decrease in high-density lipoprotein, the "good" cholesterol. These changes often are temporary. Because their job is to make the heart lazy and slow, beta blockers ensure the hands, feet (reason for coldness) and brain get blood and receive less oxygen! (see: *WebMD.com* or *MayoClinic.com*)

You can avoid dangerous drugs and maintain healthy blood pressure at the same time. See if changes in your diet and physical activity are enough to improve heart health – don't just rely on prescription drugs. Take the advice of a growing legion of progressive medical practitioners who treat high blood pressure without dangerous drugs! Doctors like Alexander Leaf of Harvard Medical School, and William Roberts, editor of *The American Journal of Cardiology*, have recommended making lifestyle changes rather than drug prescriptions for high blood pressure patients!

What is Metabolic Syndrome?

Metabolic Syndrome, also known as Syndrome X or Dysmetabolic Syndrome, refers to a cluster of metabolic risk factors that can lead to heart disease (*WebMD.com*). When a person has these risk factors together, there is a greater chance of cardiovascular problems because of the *combination of risk factors.*

Metabolic Syndrome is a serious health condition that affects about 35% of adults and places them at a higher risk of cardiovascular disease, diabetes, stroke and diseases related to fatty buildups in artery walls.

The main features of Metabolic Syndrome include: insulin resistance, high blood pressure, abnormal cholesterol, and an increased risk for clotting. The underlying causes of Metabolic Syndrome are obesity, being overweight, physical inactivity and genetic factors.

The Risk Factors of Metabolic Syndrome

Metabolic Syndrome occurs when a person has three or more of the following measurements:

- **Abdominal obesity:** a waist circumference over 40 inches in men and over 35 inches in women
- **Cholesterol panel with triglyceride levels of:** 150 mg/dl or above
- **HDL ("good") cholesterol:** 40 mg/dl or lower in men and 50 mg/dl or lower in women
- **Systolic blood pressure (top number) of:** 130 mm Hg or greater
- **Diastolic blood pressure (bottom number) of:** 85 mm Hg or greater
- **Fasting blood glucose of:** 100 mg/dl or above
- **Insulin resistance or glucose intolerance** (the body can't properly use insulin or blood sugar)

You can reduce your risks of Metabolic Syndrome significantly by: reducing your weight; increasing your physical activity; eating a heart-healthy diet that's rich in fiber including: beans, legumes, whole grains, nuts, fruits and vegetables; and monitoring your blood glucose, blood cholesterol count and blood pressure.

17 Deadly Daggers of Arterial Disease

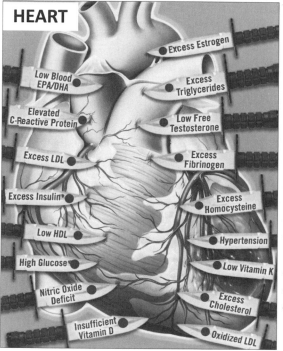

HEART

- Excess Estrogen
- Low Blood EPA/DHA
- Excess Triglycerides
- Elevated C-Reactive Protein
- Low Free Testosterone
- Excess LDL
- Excess Fibrinogen
- Excess Insulin
- Excess Homocysteine
- Low HDL
- Hypertension
- High Glucose
- Low Vitamin K
- Nitric Oxide Deficit
- Excess Cholesterol
- Insufficient Vitamin D
- Oxidized LDL

- Low Blood EPA/DHA
- Elevated C-Reactive Protein
- Excess LDL (Bad Cholesterol)
- Excess Insulin
- Low HDL (Good Cholesterol)
- High Glucose
- Nitric Oxide Deficit
- Insufficient Vitamin D
- Excess Estrogen
- Excess Triglycerides
- Low Free Testosterone
- Excess Fibrinogen
- Excess Homocysteine
- High Blood Pressure (Hypertension)
- Low Vitamin K
- Excess Cholesterol
- Oxidized LDL

Image is from: Sept. 2010, pg. 16
Life Extension Magazine

 43

This heart depicts daggers aimed at a healthy heart. Any one of these daggers would kill if thrust deep into the heart. In the real world, however, many ageing humans suffer small pricks from points of these deadly daggers over a lifetime. The cumulative dagger pricks risk effects are arterial occlusion, angina pain or acute heart attack!

Shocking Heart Facts About the #1 Killer

- *About 18.2 million adults age 20 and older have Cardiovascular Disease.*
- *One person dies every 36 seconds in the U.S. from Cardiovascular Disease.*
- *Heart disease doesn't just kill the old; 2 out of every 10 are under 65!*
- *Heart Disease is the leading cause of death for men, women, and people of most racial and ethnic groups in the United States.*
- *Heart Disease is costing United States over $219 billion every year.*

Don't let cardiovascular disease affect you! Protect your heart!
Statistics from the CDC

Our lifestyle habits, good or bad, are something we can control. – Dr. E.J. Stieglitz

Over 85% of those with hypertension can normalize blood pressure through healthier lifestyle living! If you have hypertension, then you can balance your blood pressure, glucose, leptin, and insulin levels – all at the same time – without harmful and/or ineffective medications. – LifeExtension.com

Don't Procrastinate – Improve Health Now

What kind of lifestyle changes are best? Those that instill the healthy habits we teach with The Bragg Healthy Lifestyle! A low-fat, vegetarian diet is crucial for the free flow of blood through your body. Reducing fat in your diet also stimulates weight loss, which contributes to reduced blood pressure. Make exercise a part of your daily routine and learn to breathe deeply and relax, freeing yourself of stress while filling yourself with ample fresh oxygen.

Please listen to Dr. Claude Lenfant, the longest serving Director of the National Heart, Lung & Blood Institute. He said, ***"Lifestyle changes alone can actually reverse the conditions of heart disease."*** When it comes to making the kind of changes needed for healthy and happy living, the truly important thing is making those changes happen. So don't play procrastinating games with yourself! Millions of successful Bragg students will tell you the same thing: the beginning is the most difficult. The in-between moment after you decide you want to become healthier and before you begin to act on that decision, is the hardest.

Once you dedicate your life to health you're living The Bragg Healthy Lifestyle – your Fountain of Youthfulness! Soon you will look forward with joy to your daily exercises. You will wonder how you could ever have eaten the unhealthy and unappetizing foods that once half-way sustained you. Plan, plot and follow through with The Bragg Healthy Lifestyle living. Getting started is what counts. Start Now!

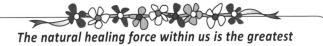

The natural healing force within us is the greatest force in getting well. – Hippocrates, The Father of Medicine

Don't procrastinate and keep waiting for "the right moment." Today – take action, plan, plot and follow through with your goals, dreams and healthy living! You will be a winner in life when you Captain your life to success!
– Patricia Bragg, Pioneer Health Crusader

Everything in excess is opposed by nature. – Hippocrates

Chapter 6

Blood – Your Precious River of Life

The body is composed of billions of tiny cells that are nourished by the blood carrying nutrients from the food we eat. As we read in the Bible, *"The life of the flesh is in the blood"* *(Leviticus 17:11).* If we can keep our body's blood in perfect chemical balance – so our vital organs and all the cells of our tissues are properly nourished – and if we keep our body's pipes open and free from corrosion, there is no reason why we can't enjoy a long lifetime of *youthful* living. Healthy blood and good circulation are the answers to a long, heart-healthy life free of premature debility and heart disease.

You can start to grasp the power you have to change your health by realizing that *all the red blood cells* in the bloodstream undergo a *complete change every 28 days.* They reproduce themselves about 12 times a year through a series of renewal processes that continue from the cradle to the grave. Our red blood cells are manufactured chiefly from the food we eat and the beverages we drink. If we put the correct nutrients into our bodies and keep our arteries, veins and capillaries clean, open and free from corrosion, we can increase our lifespan.

45

Unhealthy Foods and "Dirty" Blood Cause Illness and Premature Ageing

Many humans do not face the realities of life and live in a dream world. When you tell the average sick person that all their physical troubles are due to a "dirty, filthy bloodstream," caused by an unhealthy diet and lifestyle, often they are sensitive and insulted! They want all the modern tests and a specific diagnosis. Then they want special names and treatments given to their problems. But they still want to smoke, drink alcoholic beverages, tea, coffee, soft and cola drinks and continue eating lifeless, demineralized, devitaminized, refined, sugared, bleached, dead foods filled with harmful, lifeless calories! They want their doctor to instantly banish their aches and pains! How can their physical troubles vanish when the individual keeps breaking important health laws?

Body's Main Nourishing Arteries & Veins – A Walking, Talking, Human Miracle Machine

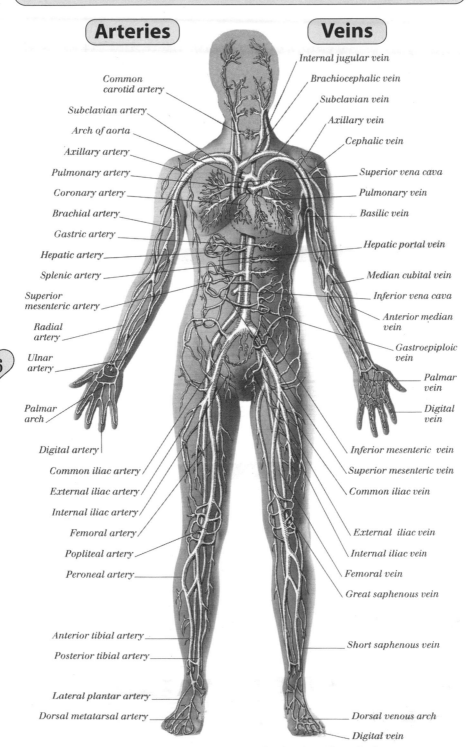

Arteries

- Common carotid artery
- Subclavian artery
- Arch of aorta
- Axillary artery
- Pulmonary artery
- Coronary artery
- Brachial artery
- Gastric artery
- Hepatic artery
- Splenic artery
- Superior mesenteric artery
- Radial artery
- Ulnar artery
- Palmar arch
- Digital artery
- Common iliac artery
- External iliac artery
- Internal iliac artery
- Femoral artery
- Popliteal artery
- Peroneal artery
- Anterior tibial artery
- Posterior tibial artery
- Lateral plantar artery
- Dorsal metatarsal artery

Veins

- Internal jugular vein
- Brachiocephalic vein
- Subclavian vein
- Axillary vein
- Cephalic vein
- Superior vena cava
- Pulmonary vein
- Basilic vein
- Hepatic portal vein
- Median cubital vein
- Inferior vena cava
- Anterior median vein
- Gastroepiploic vein
- Palmar vein
- Digital vein
- Inferior mesenteric vein
- Superior mesenteric vein
- Common iliac vein
- External iliac vein
- Internal iliac vein
- Femoral vein
- Great saphenous vein
- Short saphenous vein
- Dorsal venous arch
- Digital vein

46

Remember Your Body is A Miracle!
– Patricia Bragg, Pioneer Health Crusader

Your Bloodstream Carries Your Oxygen

Every one of the over 100 trillion cells in your body demands a continuous flow of life-giving oxygen in order to stay alive, do its job and remain healthy! Red blood cells carry this oxygen via a bloodstream teeming with life. Each of us has between 25 and 35 trillion red cells in our 5 to 6 quarts of blood – millions of cells in every drop!

We have so many of these red couriers of life and health that, in a normal healthy person, the death of 8 million red blood cells every second is not even felt! This is because, in a normal healthy person, 8 million new baby red blood cells are born into existence every second, ready to continue the work of transporting vital oxygen throughout the body.

Life Depends On Your Blood – Your River of Life

These red cell carriers of the body's oxygen are entrusted with the most important of life-sustaining jobs, but they cannot circulate and distribute their cargo on their own! They are swept along in the bloodstream – the miracle river of life. The red cells and their non-oxygen carrying siblings, white blood cells, swim downstream together in the *plasma* of your bloodstream. Plasma is practically all water; it makes up over half the volume of blood. In addition to the blood cells, plasma carries food, antibodies (for fighting off threatening, foreign intruders), hormones (for regulating body systems) and platelets (for sealing vascular breaks and removing wastes). All the wonders of human life and health depend on blood, it's absolutely essential that you live a healthy lifestyle and keep your precious bloodstream unclogged, and healthy!

47

Blood flow can also be impeded as an indirect result of inflammation. When an artery becomes inflamed, plaque becomes unstable and can rupture, causing formation of a blood clot – and a subsequent heart attack or stroke.

Your Miracle Heart propels blood through thousands of miles of blood vessels, pumping over 30 times its weight in blood each minute. Even at rest, the heart pumps over 1,800 gallons of blood daily. For all the work required of the heart, it's relatively small, about the size of a closed fist. In its pumping action, the heart delivers refreshed blood, filled with nutrients (from the food you ate) to the cells of the body through 100,000 miles of adult blood vessels to maintain your health and well-being.

Elevated C-Reactive Protein Risk Factor

C-Reactive Protein or CRP is a blood test doctors use to detect risk of heart disease, heart attack, stroke and peripheral arterial disease. CRP is a highly reactive protein that's found when there is general inflammation within the body. CRP levels are able to predict cardiovascular risk at least as well as cholesterol levels do. Excess C-Reactive Protein in blood is dangerous! A C-Reactive Protein test checks for inflammation in arteries. *Chronic inflammation* is a cause of *atherosclerosis*. Inflammation can be caused by injury to blood vessel walls, cigarette smoking, high blood pressure, etc. This can cause plaque present to rupture – triggering clots that might bring on a heart attack or stroke. Studies indicate that elevated C-Reactive Protein may even be a greater risk factor than high cholesterol in the prediction of heart attack or stroke risk.

There are risks involved when using drugs to lower C-Reactive Protein! We don't agree that people should use drugs when safer, more healthy approaches exist! There are many natural ways to lower C-Reactive Protein.

48

Safer Ways to Lower C-Reactive Proteins

- **Vitamin C:** Studies show that 1,000 mg a day reduces C-Reactive Protein just as well as some drugs.
- **Ginger:** Reduces inflammation, relaxes the muscles surrounding blood vessels and facilitates blood flow.
- **Fish Oil/Omega-3:** Reduces inflammation in blood.
- **Healthy Diet** is always safer way! Over-eating saturated fats, high-glycemic carbohydrates increases toxic CRP.

Recommended Heart Health Tests (for Adults):

- **Total Cholesterol:** 180 mg/dl or less is optimal
- **LDL Cholesterol:** 130 mg/dl or less is optimal • **HDL Cholesterol:** 50 mg/dl or more
- **Triglycerides:** 150 mg/dl or less is normal level
- **HDL/Cholesterol Ratio:** 5.0 or less • **Triglycerides/HDL Ratio:** below 2
- **Homocysteine:** 6-9 micromoles/L
- **CRP (C-Reactive Protein high sensitivity):**
  - 1 mg/L = low risk • 1-3 mg/L = average risk • over 3 mg/L = high risk
- **Diabetic Risk Tests:**
  - **Glucose:** (do 12 hour food fast) 80-100 mg/dl • **Hemoglobin A1c:** 6% or less
- **Blood Pressure:** 120/70 mmHg is good for adults

Studies show overweight individuals have elevated C-Reactive Protein Level.

Gum Disease Increases C-Reactive Protein

Numerous studies show people with gum disease double their risk of heart attack (see bottom of page 241). Acute gum disease increases amount of CRP in the bloodstream, which is a natural response to inflammation caused by injury or infection (massage gums – with apple cider vinegar on fingers massage upper gums down, lower gums massage up – don't use fluoride!) "There's evidence inflammation can be a hidden killer," said Dr. Steven Offenbacher, former President of the American Association for Dental Research regarding his abundant research on the links between gum disease and heart disease.

Gum disease can sneak up on its victims without any warning signs, according to the American Dental Association, which recommends prevention by proper diet, brushing, flossing and dental visits. Studies indicate C-Reactive Protein levels decline dramatically when periodontal disease is effectively treated.

Deadly Dangers of Elevated C-Reactive Protein

C-Reactive Protein is produced by the liver. It appears in higher amounts if there is swelling or inflammation somewhere in the body. This test can't pinpoint where the swelling is, just that there is inflammation. (*Health-and-Nutrition.org/high-c-reactive-protein*) Studies show *chronic inflammation* is directly involved in the degenerative diseases of ageing, including: cancer, dementia, stroke, visual disorders, arthritis, liver failure and heart attack. Elevated CRP levels have been called the silent killer because there are often no symptoms to indicate a problem. Fortunately a low-cost C-Reactive Protein blood test can identify if you suffer with chronic inflammation. We should all be grateful to live in an era when these vascular risk factors can be measured by a simple blood test and corrected before a major cardiovascular event manifests!

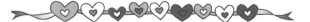

A C-Reactive Protein test measures the degree of hidden inflammation in your body. Finding out whether or not you are suffering from hidden inflammation is critical, because almost every modern disease is caused or affected by it.
– Mark Hyman, M.D., Huffpost Healthy Living • DrHyman.com

High Homocysteine Levels Cause Heart & Osteoporosis Problems

Homocysteine is an amino acid that is produced by the body, usually as a by-product of consuming meat! Amino acids are naturally made products, which are the building blocks of all the proteins in the body. High blood levels of homocysteine are a marker for heart disease, damaging cells that line blood vessel walls, setting the stage for cardiovascular disease and increasing problems with diabetes, osteoporosis and kidney diseases. When having a physical, be sure your blood panel test includes homocysteine levels. Dr. Kilmer Serjus McCully, author of *The Homocysteine Revolution* says safest and best levels are 6-8 mcm/L. Dr. Paul Dudley White agreed.

For every 10% rise in homocysteine levels, there's an equal risk of developing coronary disease and osteoporosis! In patients with heart disease, the risk of death, 4 to 5 years after diagnosis, was related to the amount of homocysteine in the plasma. Everyone produces this substance naturally, a product of protein metabolism. The homocysteine levels rise when the body is sluggish and fails to convert it to non-damaging amino acids, instead dangerously accumulating in the blood.

Studies have suggested that adequate intake of folate, vitamin B6, and vitamin B12 have resulted in lowering the homocysteine level. A healthy lifestyle menu of organic fresh fruits and vegetables offers B vitamins to help reduce high homocysteine levels.

Thank you, Dr. McCully! Your explanation of the homocysteine theory of heart disease made this a red letter day for me! – Dr. Paul Dudley White's letter to Dr. Kilmer Serjus McCully, author of "The Homocysteine Revolution"

High homocysteine blood levels (safe – 6-9 mcm/L – see chart page 48) and dietary deficiencies of vitamins (B6, B12, folic acid and CoQ10 Ubiquinol) are underlying causes of cardiovascular disease, excessive blood clotting, osteoporosis, diabetes and kidney disease. – Dr. Kilmer Serjus McCully

Be sure to get enough of the three B vitamins: Folate, B6 and B12.

You're a Self-Cleansing, Self-Repairing, Self-Healing Miracle – Please become aware of "YOU" and be thankful for all your blessings that take place daily! – Patricia Bragg, Pioneer Health Crusader

Link Between Diabetes & Heart Disease

Having diabetes puts you at an increased risk for heart disease. In fact, two out of three people with diabetes die from heart disease or stroke. Over time, high blood glucose levels damage nerves and blood vessels, leading to complications that can cause a variety of serious illnesses, including America's #1 killer – heart disease.

Researchers found when blood sugars are abnormally high, they activate a biological pathway that causes a condition called cardiac arrhythmia – irregular heartbeats that are linked to heart failure. Also, high glucose in the bloodstream damages the arteries, causing them to become stiff and hard! Fatty material building up on the inside of these blood vessels can block blood flow to the heart or brain, leading to a heart attack or stroke. Uncontrolled diabetes can eventually lead to other health problems, such as: vision loss, kidney failure, and amputations. See web: *diabetes.niddk.nih.gov*.

What You Can Do to Lower Your Heart Risk

51

You can lower your risk by keeping your blood glucose (also called blood sugar), blood pressure, and blood cholesterol close to the recommended target range – see *"Recommended Heart Health Tests"* chart bottom of page 48.

Even though the statistics may point to an increased risk of developing heart disease if you have diabetes, there's a lot you can do in terms of prevention:

• **Be active.** Aim for about 30 minutes of exercise most days (see pages 89-98). Walking is the king of exercise!

• **Eat a heart-healthy diet.** Reduce consumption of high-fat and cholesterol-laden foods such as fried foods and eggs, and eat more high-fiber foods, including whole grains, organic vegetables and fruits (see pages 136-138).

• **Lose weight**, if you're overweight (see pages 64-69).

• **Keep blood cholesterol levels within target ranges.**

• **Keep your blood glucose level within target range.**

• **Maintain optimal blood pressure level**, preferably 120/70 (see chart on page 48 for all blood test levels).

• **Quit smoking!** (see pages 84-88).

Chronic Inflammation and Heart Disease*

The discovery that inflammation in the artery wall is a real cause of heart disease is leading to a paradigm shift in how heart disease and other chronic ailments should be treated. Despite facts that 25% of the population takes expensive statin medications and we have reduced the fat content of our diets, more Americans will die this year of heart disease than ever before.

Statistics from the American Heart Association show that some 121 million Americans currently suffer from heart disease; 34 million have diabetes and 88 million have pre-diabetes. These disorders are affecting younger and younger people in greater numbers every year (pages 59-62). *"Hidden chronic inflammation is at the root of all illness including conditions like: heart disease, obesity, diabetes, dementia, depression, cancer, even autism."*

Without chronic inflammation being present in the body, then cholesterol cannot accumulate in the walls of the blood vessels and cause heart disease and strokes. Without inflammation, cholesterol would move freely throughout the body as nature intended.

52

What Causes Chronic Inflammation?

Inflammation does have a positive role to play. It is your body's natural defence against foreign invaders such as bacteria, toxins or viruses. The cycle of inflammation is highly effective in how it protects your body from these bacterial and viral invaders. However, *when we chronically expose the body to injury by toxins or foods the human body was never designed to process, "chronic inflammation" occurs*. What are the biggest culprits? The overload of simple, highly processed carbohydrates (white sugar, white flour and all the products made from them) and the excess consumption of omega-6 vegetable oils like soybean, corn and sunflower that are found in many processed foods (see page 144 for list of "Foods to Avoid"). **These foods have been slowly poisoning almost everyone.**

Dr. Dwight Lundell – Retired Heart Surgeon and Past Chief of Staff and Chief of Surgery at Banner Heart Hospital in Arizona and author of "The Cure for Heart Disease."

Chronic Inflammation & Blood Sugar

When we consume simple carbohydrates such as white sugar or white flour, our blood sugar levels rise rapidly! In response, the pancreas secretes insulin, which drives sugar into each cell where it is stored for energy. If the cell is full and does not need glucose, it is wisely rejected to avoid extra sugar gumming up the works.

When your full cells reject the extra glucose, blood sugar rises producing more insulin and then glucose converts to stored fat! Blood sugar is controlled in a very narrow range. *Extra sugar molecules attach to a variety of proteins that in turn injure blood vessel walls. This repeated injury day after day to blood vessel walls sets off toxic inflammation in your delicate blood vessels.*

Do You Have Chronic Inflammation?

How can you determine if you might have toxic chronic inflammation, especially since many "symptoms" are silent? One blood test used is the C-Reactive Protein (CRP) test, which measures a protein found in your body that signals responses to any forms of inflammation.

Another test that can be effective, depending on the severity of the disease, is an ESR (sed rate) test. Sed rate, or Erythrocyte Sedimentation Rate is a blood test that can reveal inflammatory activity in your body. A sed rate test isn't a stand-alone diagnostic tool, but it may help your doctor diagnose or monitor the progress of an inflammatory disease, (such as rheumatoid arthritis) which checks for non-specific indicators of inflammation.

You can use a fasting blood insulin level, although this test is typically used for diabetes. It's also a marker for inflammation as the higher your insulin levels are, the higher your levels of inflammation tend to be (web: *mercola.com*).

Start fasting 11 hours every night: your body needs this break to run and repair your metabolic functions. Stop eating by 7 p.m. to 6 a.m. This will help you in lowering blood sugar preventing inflammation and cell ageing.

As of 2021 it's estimated that over 463 million people worldwide suffer from diabetes. Type 2 diabetes is a condition when the body doesn't produce enough insulin to maintain normal blood sugar levels, or insulin produced doesn't work properly. This condition has been linked to obesity, poor diet and sedentary lifestyles. Experts believe most cases can be prevented by a healthy lifestyle.

Getting the Body Back into Healthy Balance

Dr. Mark Hyman (*DrHyman.com*) and Dr. Mercola (*Mercola.com*) recommend the following simple effective ways to achieve balance and reduce your inflammation:

1. Eat Whole Foods: choose unprocessed, unrefined, whole, real foods, such as organic fruits and vegetables, whole grains, legumes, nuts and seeds (see pages 136-138).

2. Enjoy Healthy Fats: getting more omega-3 fats from olive oil, nuts and avocados (see pages 128-129 and 227).

3. Optimize your insulin levels (see list page 51).

4. Exercise Regularly: regular exercise helps reduce inflammation. It also improves your immune function, strengthens cardiovascular system, corrects and prevents insulin resistance, and is key for improving your mood and erasing effects of stress! In fact, regular exercise will improve health in virtually ALL areas of your life. Now get busy moving, exercising, living healthy! (see pages 89-98).

5. Make sure your waist size is normal: Women with a waist measurement over 35" and men over 40" may have high inflammation (see page 67-69).

6. Relax your whole body: It lowers inflammation, also practice yoga and meditation, breathe deeply, read, take a relaxing hot shower or bath (see pages 79-81).

7. Avoid Allergens: find out what you're allergic to and stop eating those foods (see Dr. Coca's Pulse Test and the list of "Most Common Food Allergies" page 145).

8. Heal Your Gut: take pro-biotics. Bone broth is a wonderful source of gelatine and collagen, which is beneficial for promoting digestion and supporting a healthy gut barrier. You may also try Lemon & Ginger Tea.

9. Supplements: take multi-vitamin/multi-mineral supplement, fish oil (page 227), vitamin D3 (pages 216-217) and Turmeric (with curcumin), all help reduce inflammation.

Taking steps to reduce inflammation and balance your immune system addresses the core system of the body – your precious miracle blood! It's the basis of healthy living.

Chronic inflammation is systemic – silently damaging your tissues. – Mercola.com

Chapter 7

Heart Disease in Women:
Understanding Symptoms & Risks*

Although heart disease is often thought more of a problem for men, more women than men die of heart disease each year! More than 1 in 3 female adults in the U.S. has some form of cardiovascular disease! Women are six times as likely to die of heart disease then of breast cancer. Heart disease kills more women over 65 than all other cancers combined. Very few pre-menopausal women have heart attacks, unless they smoke, have diabetes, or are on birth control pills for a long period of time. Smoking seems to be the biggest risk factor (please read pages 84-88).

Women's heart disease symptoms can vary and be very different from the symptoms in men. Often the classic signs of chest pain are not prevalent in women. Women tend to downplay their symptoms and wait longer to seek help! Plus, historically women receive less aggressive heart disease prevention and treatment. As a result, when women are finally diagnosed, they usually have more advanced heart disease, which leads to a more dire prognosis! Fortunately, women can take steps to understand their unique symptoms of heart disease and begin to reduce their risk of heart disease!

Heart Attack Symptoms Different for Women

It's easy for women to miss heart attack symptoms at the initial stages because the symptoms do show up differently in women than in men. In fact, the top four symptoms are often misdiagnosed. Immediate intervention can mean life or death, so it's a good idea for all women to be aware of the warning signs of heart attacks. Signs and symptoms are more subtle than the obvious crushing chest pain often associated with heart attacks. Women tend to have blockages not only in their main arteries, but also in the smaller arteries that supply blood to the heart – a condition called small vessel heart disease or *Microvascular Disease*.

For more info on heart disease in women visit these websites:
• Heart.org • GoRedForWomen.org • WomenHeart.org

Many women tend to show up in emergency rooms after much heart damage has already occurred because their symptoms are not those typically associated with a heart attack. If you experience these symptoms or think you're having a heart attack, call for emergency medical help immediately. Don't drive yourself to the emergency room.

Women's Symptoms Prior to Heart Attack:

Women will experience different symptoms of a heart attack. Some women experience several symptoms, while others show all symptoms. As with men, the most common heart attack symptom in women is chest pain or discomfort. But there are women who show no symptoms before their heart attack. The sooner you recognize and take appropriate action, the better.

Here are major symptoms in women *preceding a heart attack:*

- Shortness of Breath
- Sleep Disturbance
- Flu-like Symptoms
- Unexplained Sweating
- Unusual fatigue
- Indigestion
- Pain in neck, jaw, upper back, chest
- Nausea
- Heartburn
- Anxiety
- Dizziness

Knowing these symptoms beforehand, may help women and their doctors identify the early warning symptoms of a heart attack so they can better prevent the attacks. Don't be shy – it's your heart and your life!

Angina – an Underlying Heart Problem

Angina is chest pain or discomfort that occurs when an area of your heart muscle doesn't get enough oxygen-rich blood. Angina itself isn't a disease. It's a symptom of *Coronary Artery Disease (CAD),* the most common type of heart disease. Angina may feel like pressure or squeezing in your chest or it may feel like indigestion. You may have pain in your shoulders, arms, neck, jaw or back. Nausea, fatigue, shortness of breath, sweating, light-headedness or weakness also may occur.

Women are at serious risk of heart disease, especially after menopause. In fact, coronary-artery disease is the leading killer of women over 65. Five times more women die of heart disease than of breast cancer. Vital statistics show 53% of women still die of atherosclerotic vascular disease (includes coronary-artery disease, stroke, aneurysms, etc.) compared to 42% of men dying of these causes.

Signs & Symptoms During Heart Attack:

Here are major acute symptoms *during a heart attack* in woman:

- Shortness of breath
- Cold sweat
- Dizziness
- Nausea/Vomiting
- Unusual Fatigue
- Weakness
- Pain that runs along neck, jaw, upper back or chest

What To Do Fast During Possible Heart Attack

If you experience any of the above signs or symptoms:

- Do not wait to call for help. Dial 9-1-1. Make sure to follow operator's instructions and get to hospital immediately.
- Survive, don't drive – do not drive yourself to the hospital.
- Try to stay as calm as possible and take deep, slow breaths while you wait for the emergency responders.

Women's Risk Factors are Different

What is a risk factor? Risk factors are conditions or habits that make a person more likely to develop a disease. They can also increase the chances that an existing disease will get worse. When it comes to heart disease, there are many health and lifestyle factors that can influence your risk. Be aware of your risk factors – take them seriously. The actions you take now to lower your risk may just save your life.

Although traditional risk factors for heart attack – such as high cholesterol, high blood pressure and obesity – affect women and men, there are other factors that play a bigger role in development of heart disease in women.

- **Metabolic Syndrome** – a combination of fat around the belly, high blood pressure, high blood sugar and high triglycerides – has greater impact on women (see page 42).
- **Mental stress and depression** affect women's hearts.
- **Smoking** is greater risk factor in women (see pages 84-88).
- **Diabetes and being physically inactive**
- **Low levels of estrogen after menopause** pose a large risk factor for developing cardiovascular disease (see next page).

A study found women with the lowest DHEA blood levels, more than doubled their rate of dying from coronary artery disease. Taking appropriate DHEA supplements may help you achieve higher levels.

Menopause, Estrogen & Cardiovascular Health

Estrogen keeps blood vessels flexible so that they can relax and expand to accommodate blood flow. During menopause, however, estrogen levels drop, raising women's risk of heart disease (and giving hot flashes!). The level of fats in the bloodstream increase while the walls of the blood vessels collect an increased level of plaque. What's more, the weight gain that often goes hand in hand with menopause also increases the risk of heart disease, according to Northwestern Memorial Hospital. Josh Trutt, M.D., a healthy ageing expert in New York City states, *"the more time that goes by without estrogen in the body, the more plaque that builds up in a woman's arteries."*

Recovering From A Heart Attack

Chances of recovery improve dramatically if you make necessary changes in your life. Lifestyle changes include:

- Healthy eating plan
- Reduce stress
- Be physically active
- Relax
- Quit smoking
- Lose weight
- Control diabetes
- Reduce anger

You have to put yourself, your health and your heart's recovery first above all else. It must become your number one priority. If you find this difficult, you are not alone. Many of us have spent our whole lives putting the needs of others ahead of our own.

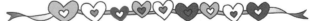

Women's Health Initiative showed that the chances of suffering a heart attack, stroke or life-threatening blood clot increase within the first two years of taking Hormone Replacement Therapy (HRT).

Research by the National Institutes of Health (NIH) indicates that women often experience new or different physical symptoms as long as a month or more before actually experiencing a heart attack.

Women should know that not every heart attack symptom is going to be the "left arm hurting". Be aware of intense pain in the jaw. Nausea and intense sweating are also common symptoms. 60% of people who have a heart attack while sleeping do not wake up. Pain in the jaw can wake you from a sound sleep! Be careful, be aware. The more you know, the better your chance to survive. – see web: doctoroz.com

Chapter 8

Heart Disease and Children

Early Lifestyle Can Trigger Obesity & Disease!

Lifestyle triggers obesity in kids. Many young people are not physically active on a regular basis and physical activity declines dramatically during adolescence. Regular physical activity in childhood and adolescence improves strength and endurance, helps build a healthy heart, bones and muscles, helps control weight, reduces anxiety and stress and increases self-esteem! It also helps normalize blood pressure and cholesterol levels.

A positive self-image is important for weight control. There are many ways you can help an overweight child regain control of their own weight. Turn off the TV, and video games, put down the electronic devices and encourage more physical activity; sports, handball, basketball, martial arts, swimming, trampolining, jump rope, tennis, etc. Teach nutrition and healthy eating practices, not only by making healthy meals, but by your example – eat the right foods and avoid fast foods, high sugar snacks, sodas and desserts altogether. Substitute healthy fresh fruit snacks and raw veggie stick snacks. Eat slowly and chew each mouthful thoroughly. Don't overeat! The Bragg Healthy Lifestyle books inspire and help establish life-long healthy habits for all ages, especially children! Exercising, eating healthy foods, and a weekly fast day all help teach children early prevention to keep healthy and stay fit for life!

59

Americans overeat, starting in childhood confirms Mayo Clinic Analysis. They ingest more calories than their body utilizes – jeopardizing health and longevity.

A study published in the "Archives of Internal Medicine" found that eating the equivalent of a quarter-pound of hamburger daily for ten years, gives men a 27% higher risk of dying of heart disease and 22% risk of dying of cancer; while women had a 50% higher risk of dying of heart disease!
Follow The Bragg Healthy Lifestyle to protect your precious heart!

I am beginning to learn that it is the sweet, simple things of life which are the real ones after all. – Laura Ingalls Wilder, Author

Childhood Obesity – Huge Growing Problem

A growing concern is the increase in obesity among children and adolescents. The problem of childhood obesity is a grave one, that can have many lasting effects on one's emotional and physical health!

Apple A Day Helps Keep Doctor Away!

High Fat, High Sugar, Salty, Fast Foods, Junk Foods Promote Obesity

It is estimated that about a third of all U.S. children are at risk for developing Type 2 Diabetes in their lifetimes. Overweight children are at risk for having high levels of cholesterol, blood pressure and insulin, making them excellent candidates for conditions like heart disease, diabetes and cancer. For obese children, they can develop heart disease, gallbladder and liver disease, diabetes, and sleep apnea. A report documented nine cases over the course of 11 years in children as young as 12 years old having had rare heart attacks, which stated, *"this is an under-recognized problem*! Pediatricians need to understand that this is a true and real condition!" Don't just push aside any child that is complaining of chest pain.*

According to research conducted by the Centers for Disease Control, studies show among children between the ages of 6 and 11, the rate of obesity has tripled. More than a third of young people do not regularly engage in vigorous physical activity. Daily participation in school P.E. classes has dropped across the United States.

A heart attack in children is typically a chest crushing-type pain that radiates to arm, jaw or neck – similar to adults' symptoms. – CBS News

People who eat fast food twice a week and spend 2 and a half hours or more a day watching T.V. have triple the risk of obesity when compared to those who eat out once a week or less and watch no more than an hour and a half of TV.

A major factor in the obesity epidemic is kids being a primary target for processed food and beverage manufacturers. The processed food industry has created an entire field of science devoted to creating flavors and textures children will crave. Junk food addiction is very real! Children become obese because they get addicted to processed foods that create metabolic havoc. – mercola.com

60

Why Are So Many Children Overweight?

The answer is painfully obvious, children overeat sugar, fat, salty junk foods and exercise too little. Children often come home from school and sit and watch TV ads* for high fat, sugar foods. A double whammy! The average American child spends from 2 to 4 hours a day watching TV, playing video games using electronic devices – time that could be spent in healthy physical activity. Remove TV, phones and computer from bedrooms, limit mesmerizing screen time.

Studies Show That Teenagers Now Susceptible to Heart Disease

A study by Nutritional biochemist, Dr. T. Colin Campbell of Cornell University found that one out of two children born today will develop heart disease, and a new study from the American Heart Association Scientific Sessions (*AmericanHeart.org*), shows that heart disease actually begins developing early in childhood. Fatty deposits in coronary arteries begin appearing by age 3, in children who partake in a typical American diet of processed foods laden with fats. By age 12, nearly 70% of children have advanced fatty deposits, and by age 21, the early stages of heart disease is evident in virtually all young adults! Dr. John Knowles, of the Rockefeller Foundation, cited 99% of all children are born healthy, yet are made sick as a result of their lifestyle eating habits! Studies also find "adult" diseases are related to what we eat throughout our early years in life. The tender years of childhood should be the healthiest of all: bones are strong, hair is thick, liver and endocrine glands are functioning to full capacity, and they should have inexhaustible energy. Yet, their bodies are being fed hamburgers full of steroids, antibiotics, hormones and chemicals; milk that is often indigestible which can cause earaches, colds, mucus allergies, asthma and many health problems. – Study from: *AmericanHeart.org*

61

Children ages 8-12 saw an average of 21 TV ads each day for candy, snacks, cereal and fast foods over (7,600 ads yearly), according to a Kaiser Family Foundation Study.

Childhood obesity has both immediate and long-term effects on health and well-being. – www.cdc.gov/healthyyouth/obesity/facts.htm

Choose A New Healthier Direction

Change your bad lifestyle habits for good ones. Of course, it's easier for kids to make better choices if they see their parents doing the same! So make a plan to help your entire family choose a new, healthier direction! After all, getting a late start on the right path beats staying on the wrong one. Follow these Bragg Healthy Lifestyle tips:

Get more exercise. By taking just one of those hours spent in front of the TV or computer each day and spending it on something that gets the blood flowing, kids (and adults) can dramatically improve blood pressure, cholesterol, and sensitivity to effects of insulin.

Eat mindfully. A child who learns to see food as fuel and not emotional compensation can start to make better choices at all meals. For example: selecting complex instead of simple carbs (such as whole-grain instead of white bread, and brown rice instead of white); increasing fiber intake with more beans, fruits, and vegetables; choosing "healthy" fats like olive oil and nuts; and avoiding too many empty calories from soda and sweets.

62

Fiber supplements. If your child is not getting enough fiber through salads and their foods, a fiber supplement (psyllium husk tab or powder) provides an added boost to help elimination and reduce LDL cholesterol in blood.

Not smoking. Smoking is the worst thing young people can do, it greatly increases your child's risk for developing heart disease, lung cancer and brain fog!

Here's a great thing kids can learn about cause-and-effect: they have the power to positively influence many health outcomes. Eating right and staying active are two ways they can help ensure a healthier tomorrow.
– Steven Dowshen, M.D., podiatric endocrinologist, Nemours Alfred I. duPont Hospital for Children, Delaware.

If I were to name the three most precious resources of life, I would say books, friends and nature; the greatest of these, at least the most constant and always at hand is Mother Nature and God. – John Burroughs

In a Harvard Alumni Study, walking two miles a day, seven days a week, produced the highest protection to stay happy and healthy and not have a heart attack!

Chapter 9

Invest in Your Body's Health

Health has sometimes been defined as *physical unconsciousness*. Not all physical unconsciousness is health, but the greatest compliment we can pay to the functioning of our body is to be unaware of it because it is running so smoothly. Most young people do not realize there is such a thing as health because when young, most have it in abundance.

With the passage of years, however, we tend to become aware, thus more *health-conscious*. The adage is so often true that says: *You spend your Health to gain your Wealth*. In later life, its reverse proves true: *You spend your Wealth to regain your Health*. The health-conscious person usually becomes so only after getting sick, and we are of the opinion that most people over 50 are a little sick. There would be no such thing as health if it were not for the lack of it. Most people begin to discover health's existence just when they need it the most. While *health consciousness* may be the result of impaired vitality, let us suggest this applies only to the common variety of health and *health consciousness*.

Invest in Your "Health Bank" for Comfort, Health Security and Happiness

Higher Health is essentially conscious or rather, it's the *conscious of its unconsciousness*. It is *health pride – something you should truly cherish*. It's a will and a desire manifestation to live a long, happy, active and healthy life.

Can you think of any greater comfort, security and happiness than that of perpetual sound health? Or that any of your loved ones need never be stricken with an early death from heart disease?

The more you praise, honor, and celebrate your life, then the more there is to be thankful for and celebrate! – Oprah Winfrey

The unexamined life is not worth living. It is time to re-evaluate your past as a guide for a bright, healthy future. – Socrates, ancient Greek Philosopher

Start Investing in Your Health Bank

Perhaps supreme super health seems *too good to be true*. Yet this ideal state of affairs is attainable by anyone willing to apply the principles of our Heart Fitness Program. It is our sincere conviction that the tragic prevalence of heart diseases, as well as many other diseases, is entirely unnecessary and is strictly within one's own control to prevent. Let health become a serious pursuit with you. The time and effort you spend following our Heart Fitness Program will be an investment in your *Health Bank*. This wise investment will bring you and your loved ones great returns in happiness and security. Always remember, *Your Health is Your True Wealth!* This teaching contained in our Heart Fitness Program – if followed faithfully and conscientiously – cannot fail to result in your acquiring and maintaining a more youthful, fit heart. Again, let us emphasize that our Heart Fitness Program does not offer a cure for heart disease, nor can it do anything until it is applied! But remember – the body can do miracles in healing itself if given a chance, as has been proven in thousands of cases.

The "Big Three" of Health and Longevity

✦ *Rule #1: Maintain a healthy weight for your body type.* Eating a fresh, vegetarian diet without sugar, dairy, processed foods, fast foods, fried foods, white flour, alcohol, soda and salt. Encourage healthy weight loss and the ability to maintain a fit and vibrant body.

✦ *Rule #2: Daily exercise is a must for a healthy heart.* Vigorous daily exercise helps you to keep your weight normal, it will also stimulate a healthier flowing blood circulation throughout your body. It helps tone your muscles and vital organs, and aids all body functions, giving you the glow of Super Health!

Idleness of mind and body is the slow burial of a living man. – Jeremy Taylor

Weight gain – eventually leading to being overweight or obesity – is determined by a balance of energy. When we consume more energy – typically measured in kilocalories – than the energy expended to maintain life we gain weight. This is a called an energy surplus. When we consume less energy than we expend, we lose weight – this is an energy deficit. – ourworldindata.org/obesity

◆ *Rule #3: The most important is proper, healthy diet.* A healthy heart and body depends upon a clean, healthy bloodstream, and this depends upon the food you eat! We will discuss all of these points in detail later. When listing proper diet as point #3, we are saving the best for last. Your diet is the most important factor in controlling your ideal weight, nourishing your blood and protecting your heart from deadly-clogging cholesterol. **Proper diet will strengthen you and make your heart a** *powerful fountain of life* **and** *a fountain of eternal youthfulness.*

Your Miracle Body Constantly Works for You – And You Must Protect & Work for Your Body!

The body is constantly breaking down old bone and tissue cells and replacing them with new ones. As the body casts off old minerals and broken-down cells, it must obtain fresh food supplies of essential elements for new cells! Scientists are only now beginning to understand that various kinds of dental problems, different types of arthritis and even some forms of artery hardening are due to body imbalances of calcium, phosphorus and magnesium. Many disorders can be caused by imbalances in the ratios of these minerals to each other.

Each individual's healthy body requires a proper balance within itself of all the nutritive elements. It is just as bad for any individual to have too much of one item, as it is to have too little of another one. For instance, it takes appropriate levels of phosphorus and magnesium to keep calcium in solution so it can be formed into new cells of bone and teeth. Yet there must not be too much magnesium nor too little calcium in the diet or old bone will be taken away and new bone will not be formed. We know that diets that are unbalanced can deplete the body of essential minerals and elements.

There is truth in the saying that man becomes what he eats. – Mahatma Gandhi

We know that organic whole grains and organic produce contain fiber that's important in lowering blood cholesterol levels. Diets high in fiber also tend to be relatively low in calories. This healthy eating pattern helps keep weight down and can ward off diabetes which is a big heart disease risk (see page 51).

Diets high in meats, fish, eggs, grains and nuts and their products may provide unbalanced excesses of phosphorus which could leech calcium and magnesium from the bones, causing them to be lost in the urine.

A diet high in fats tends to increase the intake of phosphorus from the intestines relative to calcium and other minerals. Such diets can also produce a loss of body's basic minerals in the same way a high phosphorus diet does. Diets excessively high in fruits/juices may cause unbalanced excesses of fruit sugars (pre-diabetes) in the body, which also could leech calcium and magnesium from the body.

What is "Normal Weight?"

There are numerous charts, tables and statistics on the subject of normal weight for particular ages, heights, etc. These are based on averages. However, *there is no such thing as an average person.* You may use such statistics as a general guide, but they should not be applied arbitrarily to determine your exact healthiest weight.

If you give your body the proper, healthy diet and ample exercise, you will naturally attain and maintain your best personal weight! To weigh a certain number of pounds does not necessarily indicate your proper measurement of waist, hips, etc. If you are firm and healthy – without excess flab – it doesn't matter whether you weigh more or less than the chart *average* for your years and height. The important thing is to *find your own best weight as the result of proper care you give your body.* If your body is healthy, trim and fit, then your weight is normal for you. *Remember that excess flabby fat is never normal!*

Beware of Excess "Flabby" Fat

A normal amount of fatty tissue is an indication of health. But when fatty accumulations begin to bulge out here and there and destroy your youthful outlines – beware! These are danger signals warning you that it is time to take action to slim down your excess weight.

Ten Little, Two-Letter Words of Action To Say Daily:
If it is to be, it is up to me!

Excess weight invites heart attacks: It puts an undue strain on your heart and indicates you have been eating saturated fats that can line arteries with artery-clogging cholesterol. Remember excess fat is fatal to overall health and makes you more prone to body injury, accident, disease and premature death! (Re-read bottom lines of page 3.)

Your Waistline is Your Lifeline, Youth-line, Date-line and Health-line

Fat around the abdomen presents more of a heart disease risk than fat on the hips, thighs and buttocks. When you have a "spare tire" you are flirting with premature old age! You are allowing the old age cells to gather in your body.

"Visceral Fat" Linked to Heart Disease, Diabetes, Stroke & Other Chronic Diseases*

Your body has two types of fat: *visceral* and *subcutaneous*. Subcutaneous fat is found just under your skin and causes dimpling and cellulite. Visceral fat shows up in your abdomen and surrounds your vital organs including your liver, heart and muscles. Visceral fat spells trouble for your health. It drives up your risk for diabetes, heart disease, stroke, and even dementia.

If you are eating a diet that is high in white sugar and refined grains – this is the same type of diet that will also increase inflammation in your body (see pages 52-54) – as the sugar gets metabolized in fat cells, fat releases surges in *leptin*. Over time, if your body is exposed to too much leptin, it will become resistant to the leptin (just as your body can become resistant to insulin).

When you become *leptin-resistant*, your body can no longer hear the messages telling it to stop eating and burn fat – so it remains hungry and stores more fat. Leptin-resistance also causes an increase in visceral fat, sending you on a vicious cycle of hunger, fat storage and an increased risk of heart disease, diabetes and more.

Recent studies show people with large waistlines have shorter lifespans!

*Excerpt From Dr. Mercola article • www.mercola.com

67

How You Can Stop "Visceral Fat"

Avoid eating pro-inflammatory foods such as white sugar, soda, alcohol, bread (refined grains) and trans fats (for list of "Foods to Avoid" see page 144). Foods that will reduce inflammation are fruits and vegetables, omega-3 fats like fish oil and certain spices like ginger.

Exercise is critical! Exercise is one of the best weapons to fight visceral fat – it drastically reduces visceral fat and lowers inflammation. One study found that volunteers who did not exercise had an 8.6% increase in visceral fat after 8 months, while those who exercised the most lost over 8% of their visceral fat during that time.

So whether you are thin or carrying excess belly fat, embarking on a healthy nutrition plan and exercise program will do wonders for your future health and longevity.

Be Your Body's Health Captain

For a strong, healthy heart you must faithfully practice Health Mindedness! In your mind's eye see yourself as you wish to be – strong, healthy and youthful. A person in charge of his body is not a slave to unhealthy lifestyle habits!

Free yourself from bondage of these killing habits:
- ✦ "I will not use tobacco."   ✦ "I will not over-eat."
- ✦ "I will not consume sugar."   ✦ "I will not use salt."
- ✦ "I will not drink coffee, black tea, soda and alcohol."
- ✦ "I will not clog my arteries with saturated fats."

For Better Health Break All Your Bad Habits

Habits that destroy the health of your body must be broken with strong willpower! Say to yourself repeatedly and believe it, that your intelligent mind will health captain your body towards super health! Let no person or circumstances break your iron willpower! You must do your own thinking! You can and will control your own mind, body and health.

The alcohol habit is the most harmful to the body and heart and must be stopped! The CDC states excessive alcohol consumption is third largest cause of death, after smoking and obesity!

Coffee and Non-Herbal Teas are Drugs

Coffee is a harmful stimulant to the heart. It contains the drug caffeine which makes the heart beat faster and puts it under an undue, unhealthy strain! Coffee also contains tars and acids which are injurious to the heart, blood vessels and other tissues. These same agents are also present in decaffeinated coffee. Don't drink coffee – it has no nutrients and no vitamins or minerals! Don't contaminate blood with toxins – black teas also contain tannic acid that's used to cure shoe leather!

Study Shows Cola Drinks Toxic To Body

What do cola drinks contain? Three toxic stimulants and carbonated water! Colas contain caffeine, phosphoric acid and refined white sugar (also some diet colas contain toxic aspartame, see page 70); all are toxic empty calories without any health value. They also contain carbonated water, which irritates the kidneys and liver! *Studies say: Don't drink colas or any sodas – and don't let your children ruin their health with these drinks!* According to the Center for Science in the Public Interest, an average American teenager is drinking twice as much soda pop as back in 1974. One-fourth of teenagers get 25% or more of their calories from soda, which is filled with sugar. In fact, teens consume 2-3 times as much sugar than U.S. government guidelines! Another study links increased soda consumption to heart disease, diabetes, obesity, kidney stones and calcium deficiency.

69

Alcohol is a Depressant and a Killer!

Alcohol, generally considered a stimulant, is actually a depressant. It dilates the blood vessels, in time breaking the tiny capillaries, especially of the nose, cheeks, neck and ankles (example: red, swollen nose of hard drinkers). Alcohol is also a relaxant, that dulls and paralyzes the brain. The drinker loses good judgement and control of the body and the brain becomes confused. This is therefore

A fit, youthful body must be faithfully maintained. This requires proper care of your priceless human machine. The rewards are well worth the effort! If you find fatty tissue accumulating, increase your exercise and reduce the quantity of food you eat and fast one day a week (see pages 163-170 for more on fasting).

the cause of millions of car accidents, crimes, killings, rapes, fights and unnecessary deaths. *Drinking alcohol is so dangerous, and certainly an unhealthy way to relax!*

The chief toxic effect of alcohol is on the brain and nervous system! Alcohol *burns up* by depleting the body of vitamin C and also B (the essential nerve vitamin). This, in combination with capillary dilation, can lead to brain hemorrhaging – which in turn, can lead to paralysis. Medical research has shown that the boisterous actions, loud speech, joviality, bravado and *devil-may-care* attitude of the alcoholic are actually the beginning paralysis of certain parts of the brain! Visit: *alcoholics-anonymous.org*

Stay away from alcohol!! It is nothing but *empty calories*. The *numbing effect of alcohol* on the pain centers of the brain and nervous system is a *special danger to anyone with a heart condition*. Without being alert to Mother Nature's warning signal – pain – a heart attack, which could be averted when action is taken, may prove fatal!

Say "No" to Self-Drugging TV Ads!

If you try the TV drugs for yourself, the side-effects and long-term results could be serious! Even though constant TV ads tell us what to take to solve aches, pains, upset stomach, insomnia, etc., plus side-effects, everyday more than 36 million people take over-the-counter and prescription drugs for pain relief, headaches, heartburn, arthritis, etc. with nearly 25% exceeding the recommended dosage. However, there is an increased risk of gastrointestinal complications ranging from stomach pain to ulcers, hemorrhage, and severe and potentially deadly gastrointestinal problems. Each year, the side effects of long-term drug use cause nearly 103,000 hospitalizations and 16,500 deaths by some estimates.

Beware of Toxic, Deadly Aspartame and Chemical Sugar Substitutes!

Although its name sounds "tame," this deadly neurotoxin is anything but! Aspartame is an artificial sweetener (over 200 times sweeter than sugar) made by Monsanto Corporation and marketed as "Nutrasweet,"

"Equal," "Spoonful," and countless other trade names. Although aspartame is added to over 9,000 food products, it is not fit for human consumption! This toxic poison changes into formaldehyde in the body and has been linked to migraines, seizures, vision loss and symptoms relating to Lupus, Parkinson's Disease, Multiple Sclerosis and other health destroying conditions. Besides being a deadly poison, aspartame actually contributes to weight gain by causing a craving for carbohydrates. A study of 80,000 women by American Cancer Society found those who used this toxic "diet" sweetener actually gained more weight than those who didn't use aspartame products.

High Fructose Corn Syrup (HFCS), is a highly toxic processed sugar that contains similar amounts of unbound fructose and glucose. What makes HFCS unhealthy is that it is metabolized to fat in your body far more rapidly than any other sugar. It is a primary factor behind a number of health epidemics, including obesity, diabetes and heart disease. For a better sugar substitute use Stevia see page 143.

Watch Out for Hidden Sugars in Food Products

Food labelers often hide sugars in their products by calling them by other names. They also use more than one kind of sugar, so that sugar will not have to be listed first, as the most common ingredient. In a list of ingredients, sugar can often be called: corn syrup, corn sweetener, high fructose corn syrup, dextrose, fructose, glucose, sorbitol, mannitol, barley malt, grape sweetener, sorghum, lactose and maltose. If even two of these "hidden" sugars are listed as the third and fourth ingredients, it may be that sugar is actually the greatest ingredient in the product. (Healthy Heart Handbook – Dr. Neal Pinckney)

The Highway to Higher Health and Happiness

Super Health and Happiness! To us, these seem inseparable. Our motto: *To make my body a temple pure, wherein I live serene.* Promoting the welfare of our hearts and bodies is a loving, religious task. By *Health* we don't mean the everyday variety that consists of *not being sick.* We are referring to what we call *Higher Health* – a sense of amazing well-being that makes a person proud to say with gusto, *I am feeling great today!*

We all agree that the chief aim of life is happiness! There is but one main avenue to happiness that we can recommend with confidence . . . and that is the Highway to Higher Health! Without balanced health – physically, mentally, spiritually and emotionally, it's difficult to have true happiness. The healthy ditch-digger is more in love with life than the sick, millionaire. Great health is the prime factor in attaining true happiness. Keep your body healthy and fit and your mind and heart will rejoice!

A Healthy Body and A Happy Mind

A happy and healthy body usually produces a happy, healthy mind. It by no means follows, however, that a happy mind will make a happy body. It would be glorious if the spirit could so triumph over the flesh. But alas the condition of the body usually has greater influence upon the mind, than the mind has upon the body. A person with a healthy sound body and who is spiritual, is seldom miserable, but it's rare for a sick, unhealthy person to be totally happy.

Research on a group of businessmen found that those who had a spiritual connection – attended church or believed in a higher power – had fewer heart problems than those who had no spiritual connection! (see page 78)

It's Never too Late to Learn and Improve

Men and women today are slowing down the ageing process by living healthier lives. The human structure is mechanically adapted for full energies and activities at 70, 80, 90 and older – clearly proven by the increased number of people worldwide who are healthy, clear of eye and keen of mind as they enter their golden years. If you want to get maximum joy out of life, start perfecting your human temple!

This is why we are Health Nutritionalists and Physical Fitness Crusaders. Happiness is largely dependent upon the care we give our bodies. Through harmony of flesh, we achieve the exultation of spirit! Mental serenity is profoundly physical in its source. Through the purification of our body's living tissues we attain a balanced life of supreme health! Let's therefore put health of our heart, body and soul first before everything, as everything else depends upon this!

Chapter 10

Doctor Human Mind & Emotions
The Effects of Stress & Anger

A Sound Mind in a Sound, Healthy Body

Shakespeare, almost four hundred years ago, anticipated the dominant psychology of our time when he said, *It is the mind that makes a body rich.* It's true that the mind guides the body. Likewise, the body helps the mind and links us to the Infinite Spirit of Life! When we are truly healthy, we are brim full in body, mind and spirit.

Our body relates us to the Universe in which we live – the Earth. We are related to Mother Earth through the food we eat, the water we drink, the air we breathe and the sunshine that warms us with its all-pervading power. All are essential for a healthy body and to the continuance of our life! We need all these nurturing things in as pure a form as Mother Nature and God have provided them, without depleting or denaturing them.

73

The food we eat is related to our daily health. Our bloodstream's system carries essential nutrients that provide the energy and vitality for the functioning of every part of the body. What we eat at this hour today will be nourishment in our cells within 24 hours.

If we eat organic foods as Mother Nature prepares with her own unmatched chemistry and without losing essential elements – then it will meet our requirements for the growth, health and chemical balance of our body. It will build a powerful, long lasting, strong heart for you. It will give you an alert and active mind. Healthy foods will add life to your years – and years to your life! When a sick person constantly convinces himself that he will never get well, it becomes almost certain that his negativity and troubles will carry him to the grave.

Give me the Serenity to accept what cannot be changed; the Courage to change what can be changed; and the Wisdom to know the difference.

"Read uplifting books and turn off the news. Just smiling can enhance your mood and health." – Kenneth R. Pelletier, Ph.D, M.D., Professor at UC San Francisco

Control Your Negative & Positive Thoughts!

Think of your thoughts as powerful self-talk magnets with the ability to attract (positive) or repel (negative) according to the way used. A majority of people lean either to positive or negative mentally. The positive phase is constructive and goes for success and positive achievements, while the negative side of life is destructive, leading to futility and failure. It is self-evident it is to our advantage to cultivate a positive, healthy, mental attitude. With patience, persistence and living The Bragg Healthy Lifestyle this can be accomplished!

Negative Emotions Bad for Health & Body

There are many negative and destructive forms of thought which react in every cell in your body! The strongest is *fear*, and its child, *worry* – along with *depression, anxiety, apprehension, jealousy, ill-will, envy, anger, resentment, vengefulness and self-pity*. All of these negative thoughts bring tension to the body and mind, leading to waste of energy, enervation and also slow or rapid poisoning of the body. *Rage, intense fear and shock* are very violent and quickly intoxicate the whole system. Worry and other destructive emotions act slowly but, in the end, have the same destructive effect. Anger and intense fear stop digestive action, upset the kidneys and the colon causing total body upheaval (diarrhea or constipation, headaches, pains, fever, etc.).

Fear, worry and other destructive habits of thought muddle the mind! A crystal clear mind is needed to reason to your best advantage, enabling you to make sound, healthy decisions! An emotionally, upset clouded mind often makes unwise and unhealthy decisions and might be unable to reach any positive conclusions at all!

The role of the mind and emotions in our state of health is a vital one. By understanding this relationship we can play a greater role in our wellbeing.
– Mark Hyman, M.D., Huffpost Healthy Living • www.DrHyman.com

"A man is literally what he thinks.
His character being the complete sum of all his thoughts."
– Quote from "As a Man Thinketh" a literary essay by James Allen, published 1902

74

Stress & Worry Eat Away at Your Health

Stress related diseases occur world-wide. In China, heart disease and stroke are projected to increase by 73% by the year 2030 or sooner! The country will lose $558 billion to these stress-related diseases, according to the World Health Organization. As in many parts of the world, decreased physical activity and unhealthy diets are leading to obesity, increased blood pressure and cholesterol and diabetes which leads ultimately to cardiac problems.

Most humans are so full of worry that they believe they can never overcome their miseries. Worrying about a problem does not solve it – it only makes things worse.

Effects of Chronic Stress on the Heart

Although Scientists do not know yet exactly how long-term stress directly affects the human heart, they do know that it often leads to other negative behaviors such as smoking, over-eating, excessive drinking or drug use, and lack of sleep! These habits, of course, will ultimately have well-known devastating effects on your heart and many other major organs of your body.

Researchers also believe that chronic stress may directly affect your heart by creating elevated, and thus unhealthy, levels of hormones such as adrenaline and cortisol. This can cause higher blood pressure, irregular heartbeats and ultimately heart disease! Continuous stress also affects the circulatory system. The arteries tend to narrow when people are in situations of very high stress that cause increased blood pressure.

"Stress also plays a major role in your immune system, and can impact your blood pressure, cholesterol levels, brain chemistry, blood sugar levels, and hormonal balance. It can even "break" your heart, and is increasingly being viewed as a cardiovascular risk marker." – Dr. Mercola

Gloom and bleakness steals joy, energy and color from your world.
You can't save your life if you don't value it! – Heart Healthy Living Magazine

My pleasant thoughts bring me peace. – Paul C. Bragg, N.D., Ph.D.

Although everyone reacts to stress differently, evidence is clear that reducing chronic stress must be one of the most important factors to consider when building a healthy body plan. Becoming aware of your personal stress levels, and learning to control them, are among the most important positive things you can do to maintain a healthy body, heart and mind!

The symptoms of chronic stress include constant feelings of anger, guilt, fear, hostility, anxiety, and moodiness. Common stressors include conflicts with supervisors or colleagues at work; overload of expectations at work; unemployment and lack of health care; finances in general; problems in personal and family relationships and most of all – self-criticism and lowered self-esteem.

Negative Emotions Connected to Heart Disease

Emotional upheaval, whether in the form of worry, depression, or anger, can increase the risk of heart disease, heart attack and stroke, research finds.

A three year study has linked negative emotions like depression, hostility and anger – with atherosclerosis, or thickening of the inside walls of the coronary arteries. Thickening of these walls can slow or block blood flow to the heart and brain, which can lead to a heart attack or stroke. *"The current evidence suggests there is a link between negative emotions and risk for heart disease – the leading cause of death in U.S."* says Dr. Stewart. In these observational studies, the strength of the connection is comparable to other well-known cardiovascular risk factors!

"Depression can be considered an emerging risk factor for heart disease," Dr. Stewart adds. *"It can be thought of as much the same way as cholesterol or high blood pressure or smoking."* Depression has been linked with increased inflammation, as measured by markers in the blood (pages 52-53). Depression also has an effect on the immune system, which then affects heart health.
– *Journal of American Medical Association*

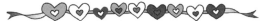

Stress puts an unhealthy strain on the heart. A UCLA study found six out of ten heart patients had constricted arteries and reduced blood flow to their heart following any emotionally charged upsets or events!

Don't Worry, Please Be Happy and Healthy!

Building positive attitude; maintaining a desire for lifelong learning and advancement; and especially constant work on reducing self-judgment and criticism, are all highly-effective at reducing stress. Daily try laughing out loud (*www.LaughterYoga.org*) and smiling at those around you. Learn to meditate or take relaxing walks; and make sure you assume responsibility for your life and what happens to you and don't blame others. This puts you in control, the Captain of your life, which helps immediately to reduce stress. Added to those efforts, of course, must be a healthy diet, regular exercise, and sufficient sleep. These are all valuable ingredients of The Bragg Healthy Lifestyle and once you make it part of your lifestyle; you will become stress-free, heart-healthy and live a longer, stronger, happier, fulfilled life.

Heart Disease and Your Personality Type

Studies have also found a strong correlation between personality traits and heart disease. The effects of stress on the heart are more prominent with those who were considered *Type-A Personalities* – defined as competitive, aggressive and impatient.

Aggressive people are also more likely to develop irregular heart rhythms and can very possibly die before reaching their 50's. High stress levels and inflammation in the walls of the coronary arteries will lead to a much higher risk of a heart attack.

Those with *Type-B Personalities* are usually more relaxed, unhurried and have fewer heart disease problems. Staying at a low stress level and being calm proves to strengthen the immune system and it puts you at a much lower risk for heart disease, so being the relaxed type B personality helps do your body and heart good.

"Being optimistic is like a muscle that gets stronger with use. Makes it easier when the tough times arrive. You have to change the way you think in order to change the way you feel."– Robin Roberts, author "Everybody's Got Something" and anchor of ABC's morning show "Good Morning America"

Smile, exercise, pray, relax, be cheerful, do yoga, and heal. – Patricia Bragg

How Spiritual Beliefs Impact Healing

Spirituality shapes life's meaning for many people. Inside that meaning lies faith, which brings about trust, positive thinking and hope. Developing and nurturing spiritual values and a deeper sense of purpose can not only keep you healthy and well, but also provide the tools to grow, develop and heal when illness arises.

Numerous research studies are finding those who have spiritual practices tend to live longer and positive beliefs can influence health outcomes. Those who are spiritual tend to have a more positive outlook on life and a better quality of life. Spirituality helps people cope with disease and face the possibility of death with peace. By cultivating a spiritual life, people are able to gain strength, hope and the ability to counteract stress, which most experts believe is at the root of almost all diseases, illnesses and health conditions. Those with a spiritual perspective also tend to believe that disease and illness are the manifestation of negative emotions and thought patterns. Feelings like resentment, criticism, guilt and fear can all lead to an imbalance in the mind and body, creating physical illness that brings with it an opportunity for self-growth. Someone who takes a spiritual approach to illness will often heal once these negative deep-rooted beliefs are addressed and overcome.

Anger & Hostility – Big Heart Disease Risks

Studies from John Hopkins School of Medicine and University of Maryland have found that irritability, hostility and dominance may cause coronary heart disease. Until recently, most research centered on the role of psychosocial factors, says Dr. Aron Siegman. The study involved 101 men and 95 women, the average age was 55 years. The research found that a full-blown outward expression of anger is a risk factor for coronary heart disease in men, and for women – subtle, indirect expressions of antagonism and anger are big risk factors! Also, expressions of irritability with anger are risk factors for coronary heart disease.

Death rates from heart disease are up four to seven times higher among people with hostile, mean attitudes, as stated by Dr. Redford Williams, Duke University Medical Center. Read his book *Anger Kills*.

Chapter 11

Doctor Deep Breathing

When You Breathe Deeply and Fully You Live Healthier and Longer

When you pump a generous flow of oxygen into your body, 100 trillion cells become more alive! This enables the four main *motors* of your body – the heart, lungs, liver and kidneys – to operate and perform better. Your miracle-working bloodstream purifies and cleanses every part of the body, including itself. This eliminates toxic wastes as Mother Nature planned, and the fuel (food) and vital oxygen are carried to every cell in your body.

With ample oxygen your muscles, tendons and joints function more smoothly! Your skin becomes firmer and more resilient and your complexion clearer and more glowing. You will then radiate with greater health and well-being for a longer, healthier life!

79

With the Bragg Super Power Breathing your brain becomes more alert and your nervous system functions better. You become free from tension and strain because you can easily take the stresses and pressures of daily living. Your emotions come under control. You feel joyous and exuberant. If negative emotions such as anger, hate, jealousy, greed or fear intrude, you can expel them by positive thinking and slow, concentrated deep breathing.

The deep breather enjoys more peace of mind and body, tranquility and serenity. In India, the great teachers practice deep, full breathing as the first essential step towards higher spiritual development! You can attain higher concentration in prayers and meditation by taking long, slow, deep breaths. Also, deep breathing stimulates your brain cells and promotes new brain cell growth.

The quality of breath should be deep, graceful, easy and efficient. – Kenneth Cohen, Health Educator

Oxygen is the vital, precious, invisible staff of life. – Paul C. Bragg, N.D., Ph.D.

Super Deep Breathing Improves Brain Power

The person who breathes deeply and fully thinks more clearly and sharply! Oxygen stimulates your brain and logic and intelligence! The more deeply and fully you breathe, the greater your power of concentration and the more your creative mind asserts itself. You will also develop greater extrasensory perception within your body, especially the brain. Scientists at the Salk Institute for Biological Studies, in La Jolla, CA, now know adults do generate new brain cells in the hippocampus, an area in the brain which is responsible for learning and memory. Deep breathing nourishes and fine-tunes the brain and entire body! (*Salk.edu*)

Read *Bragg Super Power Breathing* book. The more fully and deeply you breathe, the further you will travel to higher levels on the physical, mental and spiritual planes. Now close your eyes. Relax a few minutes while doing some slow, deep breathing! See web: *DoctorOz.com* for some relaxing breathing techniques.

The Lungs Are Nature's Miracle Breathers

Every animal extracts oxygen from the environment in which it lives. Through their gills, fish extract oxygen from water. Insects get oxygen from the air through alveoli, or air cells, in individual openings set in segments of their bodies. Worms and other invertebrates breathe through the pores of their skin. Vertebrate animals, including the human race, have those miracle mechanisms – the lungs. The mechanical equivalent would be a pair of bellows, though the lungs are far more intricate and adaptable. Human lungs are a miracle pair of conical-shaped organs composed of spongy, porous tissue. They occupy the thoracic cavity (chest) with the heart in the center, and are protected by the amazingly strong and resilient rib cage. The apex of each lung reaches just above the collar bone; the base extends almost to the waistline.

What makes up our lungs? About 800 million alveoli – air sacs of elastic tissue – which can expand or contract like tiny balloons. If these little air sacs were flattened out and laid side by side, they would cover an area of 100 square yards!

On an average day your lungs move enough air in and out to fill a medium-sized room or blow up several thousand party balloons.

Tiny capillaries (blood vessels) thread the elastic lung walls of each of the millions of air sacs and it is through these that the blood passes to discharge its load of poisonous carbon dioxide and absorb the vital, life-giving oxygen. The average person has five to six quarts of blood, which must be cleansed continually.

Air inhaled through the nose and mouth reaches the alveoli through an intricate system of tubes, beginning with the large trachea, or windpipe, which is kept rigid by rings of cartilage in its walls. The trachea extends through the neck into the chest, where it divides into two branches (bronchi), each leading into a lung cavity. Each bronchus divides into a number of successively smaller branches to bring air to every air sac.

You Have Miracle Lungs – Fill Them Up

Each lung sits perfectly enveloped in a protective elastic membrane, the pleura, whose inner layer is attached to the lung, and it's outer layer forms the lining of the thoracic cavity inside the rib cage. One end of each rib is attached to the spinal column, but the front of the rib cage is open. This allows the lungs to expand and contract. When you breathe deeply, filling every air sac, your thoracic cavity expands as your lungs fill with six to ten pints of air. This varies according to body build and size. Lungs occupy from 200 to over 300 cubic inches.

This marvelous breathing mechanism is yours for free! You are born with it. It functions without conscious effort, yet without it, you can't exist! Not even the latest inventions used by hospitals in emergencies, however ingenious, can equal the human breathing apparatus. Perhaps if human beings had to pay a fabulous price for their lungs and air, they would use them to full capacity all the time. Think of the big price you pay for only using them partially by shallow breathing. **Now, start enjoying slow, deep, relaxed breathing and feel how your body responds.**

I have shared The "Bragg Super Power Breathing" with thousands at my Sports Seminars around the world. Bragg Super Power Breathing helps make the weak strong and athletes champions. It super charges your life!
– Bob Anderson, famous stretching coach to Olympic champions • stretching.com

The Importance of Clean Air to Health

It is essential to breathe clean air – air that's as free as possible from such chemicals as smog, car exhaust, natural gas appliance fumes and the many other toxic chemical pollutants. Also, our air needs to be as free as possible from mold, dust, dust mites and their fecal matter, animal dander and pollen! Everyone's health is helped in varying degrees by clean air. It's vitally important to live and work in an area which has clean air and is free of all harmful fumes. It's also equally important to keep our homes pure, clean and free from dust, dust mites and debris! **Most people cannot be truly 100% healthy until they breathe clean air, maintain a healthy diet and live a healthy lifestyle.**

Pollutants Threaten the Lungs of All Life

Every living thing breathes. In the marvelous balance of Mother Nature, plants breathe in carbon dioxide through the pores in their leaves and give off vital oxygen – while animals inhale oxygen and exhale carbon dioxide. Both thrive in a healthy, natural balance.

82

Unfortunately, humans have played havoc with this natural balance by destroying forests and covering grass with pavement. They continue to poison our already over-burdened air with pollutants from motorized traffic and heavy industry. Wildlife, when it survives slaughter by humanity, suffocates in such polluted air. Fish die in polluted waters. How long can people survive in the midst of these environmental poisons which they continually create? This is a question of great concern to us. Read the classic book *Silent Spring* by our friend Rachel Carson, available in most libraries. If followed, her wise advice would have saved America and other nations billions of dollars and countless wildlife species! We desperately need more courageous and dedicated people like Rachel Carson to show the world the error of its ways!

Airplanes are spraying chemicals across our skies that are on OSHA hazardous list. Chemtrails have returned positive for toxic aluminum, barium, bacteria, virus and molds, causing health problems!

Your breathing habits are the first place, not the last, one should look when fatigue, disease or other evidence of disordered energy presents itself.
– Dr. Sheldon Hendler, "The Oxygen Breakthrough"

Live Longer Breathing Clean Air Deeply

We advise those who have to live or work in smoggy, polluted cities to obtain a good air filter. We especially recommend filters which contain charcoal and a high efficiency particulate HEPA air filter. The charcoal removes most of the chemicals and the HEPA filter removes most of the particles. To be effective in an average room, the flow rate through the filter should be over 200 cubic feet of air per minute. The wise motorist will also install an air filter in his car for cleaning the air while driving in air-polluted cities.

When we are born, our lungs are new, fresh, clean, and rosy in color. If we could live in a pollutant and dust-free atmosphere breathing deeply all our lives, then our lungs would remain *as good as new* for a long life of use. Yet most people abuse their lungs! Some of this comes from external causes. The lungs and skin are the only organs of the body which are directly affected by external conditions, specifically, the air breathed into the lungs!

Mother Nature provides protection against the normal amount of dust contamination: tiny nose hairs serve as filters, and moist mucus in passages leading to lungs trap dust particles that we expel through the nose or mouth. The tonsils also serve as important guards to trap germs. The lungs protect themselves remarkably well by expelling carbon dioxide through oxygenation and by discharging toxins into the blood for elimination via kidneys. *Your body is a miracle!*

Unfortunately, most civilized people today live in very unnatural conditions. Almost everywhere there are abnormal pollutants in the air we breathe, especially in urban areas. Our lungs are often overloaded with more contaminants than they can handle. These are passed into the bloodstream and to other parts of the body. Modern city dweller's lungs become brownish from car smog, soot, etc. Even in most farming areas, the lungs must contend with pollens, excessive dust, poisonous pesticides, fertilizers and other toxic chemicals. (Air purifiers and vitamin C help.)

83

The ideas that have lighted my way have been kindness, beauty and truth.
– Albert Einstein

Emphysema Smothers it's Victim

Emphysema, a killer disease from smoking, is on the rise. Medical reports show that as many as half of all American men are suffering from some degree of emphysema. In this disease, the tars, nicotine and other destructive poisons of tobacco lodge in the lungs' small air sacs, causing the sac walls to become very thin or to break down entirely. Soon the blood is no longer able to exchange poisonous carbon dioxide for life-giving oxygen. This self-destructing victim dies of oxygen starvation – being slowly smothered to death from within.

Emphysema is not a quick killer. It creeps up slowly, first with a slight cough – especially on arising. Then it attacks the smoker day and night! Slowly, air sacs are almost completely destroyed. The victim doesn't die suddenly, but lingers on steadily deteriorating. They are forced to stay near an oxygen tank because the disease is shutting off their oxygen. When the lungs can't operate any longer even with pure oxygen, the victim then dies.

Our Breath is our life! We can live days without water and weeks without food, but only minutes without air. It's the oxygen in the air we breathe that's the greatest purifying force in Mother Nature! To get this oxygen into the lungs and bloodstream, we must deeply breathe it in!

Smoking killer Tobacco is against every Natural Law! The heart needs large oxygen amounts to function. Any disease that diminishes oxygen is going to destroy the health of your heart, lungs and entire body!

Smoking Robs Your Body of Vitamin C

Vitamin C is one of Mother Nature's most essential elements for good health. In addition to its other vital functions – such as prevention of scurvy, vitamin C is also active in preventing capillaries hemorrhaging, those tiny blood vessels that directly feed the body's cells. (We take 1,000 to 3,000 mgs. mixed "C" daily, plus grapeseed extract.)

Tobacco neutralizes Vitamin C in your body, robbing you of its vital protection. Dr. W. J. McCormick – Canada's "C" Specialist – found in lab and clinical tests *smoking of a single cigarette robs the body of the amount of vitamin C contained in 1 medium sized orange.* A pack a day smoker would have to eat 20 oranges for enough vitamin "C" to accumulate in the body! Tobacco is not the only "C" thief, polluted air and foods with preservatives are as well.

When capillaries in the artery walls hemorrhage, there is additional blockage to the blood flow. When this occurs in the heart or brain, a serious clot may form. In the legs and feet serious breakdown of the capillaries may occur. Sometimes this leads to gangrene, requiring an amputation and sometimes it causes varicose veins. So you can see how essential Vitamin C is to the healthy functioning of your heart, bloodstream and entire body!

Tobacco – Deadly Enemy of Heart and Health

Whether it's cigarettes, cigars or pipes, tobacco is one of the heart's worst enemies! Here is what Dr. Lester M. Morrison, noted California Heart Specialist and pioneer of the low-cholesterol diet for the treatment and the prevention of heart disease, said about tobacco:

Tobacco is a poison! Nicotine, the main ingredient of tobacco, is a poison affecting the brain, heart and other vital organs. *The tobacco plant is directly related to the deadly nightshade family of plants. Aside from the chief poison: nicotine, there are other well-known poisons present in tobacco: arsenic and coal tar substances and the carbon monoxide when tobacco is burned.*

Dr. Morrison also said, *"Nicotine is the most noxious substance that affects the blood vessels in man. Nicotine is a powerful drug that constricts the arteries, narrowing still more the vital passageways of the blood, already clogged by other toxic residue. The tobacco smoker does double damage to his heart – first, by filling the bloodstream with the harsh poisons of tobacco and, second, by narrowing the arteries and other blood vessels, preventing a free flow of life-giving blood."*

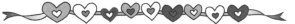

The benefits of quitting smoking start immediately! Between 5 and 10 years after quitting the risk is reduced to the same as for people who never smoked. Cutting back to fewer cigarettes a day doesn't do much to reduce the odds.

Almost 20% of all deaths from heart disease in the U.S. are directly related to cigarette smoking. That's because smoking is a major cause of coronary artery disease. – WebMD.com

Smoking Affects the Heart & Blood Vessels

Cigarette smoking causes about 1 in every 5 deaths in the United States each year. It's the main *preventable cause of death and illness* in the United States today.

Smoking harms nearly every organ in the body, including the heart, blood vessels, lungs, eyes, mouth, reproductive organs, bones, bladder, and digestive organs. The chemicals in tobacco smoke harm your blood cells. They also can damage the function of your heart and the structure and function of blood vessels. This damage increases your risk of atherosclerosis – a disease in which a waxy substance called plaque builds up in the arteries. Over time, plaque hardens and narrows your arteries. This limits the flow of oxygen-rich blood to your organs and other parts of your body. Coronary heart disease occurs if plaque builds up in the coronary (heart) arteries. Over time, this can lead to chest pain, heart attack, heart failure, arrhythmias or even death.

Smoking Major Risk Factor For Heart Disease

When combined with other risk factors such as unhealthy blood cholesterol levels, high blood pressure, and being overweight or obese, smoking further raises the risk of heart disease. Smoking is also a major risk factor for peripheral arterial disease; a condition in which plaque builds up in the arteries that carry blood to the head, organs, and limbs. People who have peripheral arterial disease are at increased risk for heart disease, heart attack and stroke.

Any amount of smoking, even light smoking or occasional smoking, damages the heart and blood vessels! For some people, such as women who use birth control pills and people who have diabetes, smoking poses an even greater risk to the heart and blood vessels.

Your lungs are precious and needed every minute of life. It's important to keep them clean and away from all smoke! – Patricia Bragg

---

The study showed most heavy smokers are snorers and are at a 1.7 times greater risk of heart disease than silent sleepers and at 2.08 times greater risk of stroke and heart disease combined. – Finnish Medical Study

---

Cigarette smoking is so widespread and significant as a risk factor that the U.S. Surgeon General has called smoking "the leading preventable cause of disease and deaths in the United States." – www.heart.org

Secondhand Smoke Also Can Harm The Heart and Blood Vessels

Secondhand smoke is the smoke that comes from the burning end of a cigarette, cigar, or pipe. Secondhand smoke also refers to smoke that's breathed out by a person who is smoking. Secondhand smoke contains many of the same harmful chemicals that people inhale when they smoke. Secondhand smoke can damage the heart and blood vessels of people who don't smoke in the same way that active smoking harms people who do smoke. Breathing secondhand smoke of others greatly increases the risk of heart attack, stroke and death.

What About Cigar and Pipe Smoke?

Researchers know less about how cigar and pipe smoke affects the heart and blood vessels than they do about cigarette smoke. However, the smoke from cigars and pipes contains the same harmful chemicals as the smoke from cigarettes. Also, studies have shown that people who smoke cigars are at increased risk for heart disease.

It's Up To You To Be Happier and Healthier!

"Actions speak louder than words and can elevate your mood if you feel depressed." Take a walk and do slow, deep breathing – it helps you sort out and solve problems. Spend time with children – it simplifies life and puts everything in perspective. Find the comics or something funny to read and laugh about. Make yourself physically smile and laugh; it opens blood vessels in the back of your head to physically lift your mood. "Choose to be happy in spite of circumstances. No one "makes" you happy – it's an attitude you self-create from within."
– *Paul C. Bragg*

Cigarette, cigar and marijuana smoke not only affects smokers. When you smoke, the people around you are also at risk for developing health problems, especially children. Secondhand smoke affects people who are frequently around smokers. It can cause chronic respiratory conditions, asthma, cancer, and heart disease. It is estimated that overly 70,000 nonsmokers die from heart disease each year as a result of exposure to secondhand smoke from others. – WebMD.com

It doesn't matter how much or how long you've been smoking – stop now and in one year your risk of heart disease will be cut by 70%.
– Dr. Daniel Levy, Framingham Heart Study Director

Quit Smoking – See Great Difference it Makes!

- **20 MINUTES AFTER QUITTING:** Your blood pressure and pulse rate start dropping to normal. The temperature of the hands and feet increases to normal.

- **8 HOURS AFTER QUITTING:** The carbon monoxide level in your blood drops to normal. The life-giving oxygen level in your blood increases to normal.

- **24 HOURS AFTER QUITTING:** You substantially lessen your chances of having a heart attack or stroke.

- **48 HOURS AFTER QUITTING:** Your nerve endings start regrowing and your ability to taste and smell is enhanced.

- **2 WEEKS TO 3 MONTHS AFTER QUITTING:** Your circulation improves. Brisk walking and exercise becomes easier. Your lung function increases as much as 30 percent.

- **1 TO 9 MONTHS AFTER QUITTING:** Coughing, sinus congestion, fatigue and shortness of breath decreases. Your lungs and body are becoming cleaner and more resistant to infection.

- **1 YEAR AFTER QUITTING:** Excess risk for coronary heart disease decreases to an amazing 50% that of a smoker's.

- **2 TO 3 YEARS AFTER QUITTING:** The risk for coronary heart disease and stroke decrease compared to those of people who have never smoked. Also less chance of osteoporosis.

- **5 YEARS AFTER QUITTING:** Lung cancer death rate for the former one-pack-per-day smoker decreases by over half. Risks of mouth and throat cancer are half those of current smokers.

- **10 TO 15 YEARS AFTER QUITTING:** Lung cancer death rate is almost that of non-smokers. Pre-cancerous cells are replaced. Risks for mouth, throat, esophagus, bladder, kidney and pancreas cancer decrease. – *Prevention Magazine • Prevention.com*

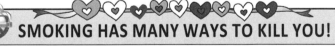

SMOKING HAS MANY WAYS TO KILL YOU!

The body has no defense against carbon monoxide produced by smoking. The coal tars in tobacco are the chief poisons responsible for cancer of the lungs, mouth and related areas of the body. It frightens us to think of what will happen in another 25 years because of excessive use of tobacco. We are convinced that every smoker (cigar and marijuana also) will develop lung, throat or some form of cancer, if heart disease doesn't kill them first.

If you smoke and already have heart disease, quitting will reduce your risk of dying from heart disease. Over time, quitting will also lower your risk of atherosclerosis and blood clots. FACT: According to the CDC, lung cancer is responsible for 28% of smoking related deaths while 43% are attributable to cardiovascular disease - primarily heart disease and strokes!

Chapter 12

Doctor Exercise

Mind Over Muscle

The saying, *"If you don't use it, you lose it"*, certainly applies to the 640 muscles of the human body. When you don't exercise regularly, your muscles lose their firm, supple tone. Over time they can become soft and flabby.

Remember that it is a lean horse that finishes and enjoys the long race! If you want a long, healthy life, keep your body trim and fit. You will be bubbling over with vitality and energy. You will be unafraid of life's challenges and be free from the fear of heart trouble and other illnesses!

Enjoy Exercising – It's Healthy and Fun!

There is great hiking near where we had a home in Hollywood, California, where Mt. Hollywood rises some 1,600 feet in famous Griffith Park. We enjoyed early morning hikes up the mountain to greet the sun rising and then would run down. Also, in Santa Barbara, we always enjoyed ocean swimming and hiking the surrounding hills.

89

We loved to walk, jog and climb mountains. We took time to walk or jog daily, or we swam, played tennis or rode our bikes. We worked out 3 times a week with a progressive weight training program, which helped keep our bones and muscles healthier and stronger.

Exercise is the greatest single factor available to us for removing any blockages and unclogging the arteries and blood vessels, and for increasing the vital flow of oxygen-enriched blood throughout the heart and body. Recent studies show that exercise can reduce the risk of developing adult-onset diabetes, as well as breast cancer. The famous Harvard School of Public Health Researchers (*www.Health.Harvard.edu*) studied a group of 70,000 women. Results: 46% lowered their risk of diabetes with daily vigorous exercising and brisk walking.

Regular exercise is a critical part of staying healthy. There are 1,440 minutes in every day. Schedule 30 of them for physical activity!

Regular aerobic exercise reduces heart attack risk by 35-55%! – Dr. Neal Pinckney

Your Heart Thrives on Exercise

Your heart needs and thrives on ample exercise! Challenging the heart through aerobic exercises such as brisk walking, running, bicycling or swimming helps it to beat more efficiently. Exercise actually expands the blood vessels around the heart, which can be a lifesaver if a blood clot latches onto one of your coronary arteries.

According to Dr. Pamela Peeke, author of *Fit to Live*, *"An out-of-shape heart can be hazardous. Fat infiltrates the heart muscle and can interfere with electrical impulses. This may cause arrhythmia, or even sudden death."* The American Heart Association (web: *Heart.org*) states that *"exercise is especially important for those with heart disease."* They recommend that you first undergo a stress test; utilizing a heart rate monitor while you work-out.

Develop Strength from the Inside Out, Not from the Outside In

Remember that from the day you were born into this world, to the day you die, your 640 muscles play an important role in everything you do. Think of it – *more than half of your body is sheer, active, working muscle!* It isn't the muscles that you see that count as much as those you don't see! Along the 30-foot gastrointestinal tract there are muscles to force food along this tube. The work of bringing adequate amounts of air into your powerful lungs also requires other strong muscles.

And above all, *the greatest muscular organ* in your body is *your heart, your number one pump*. It is the heart that pumps the blood supply into the body's 640 muscles. And the more we bring these 640 muscles into play, the better our heart, circulation, physical condition and our entire state of health will be! You have four more extra *pumps* that can also help this whole miracle process – they are your two arms and your two legs – use and exercise them!

Brisk Power Walking is the King of Exercise

Brisk power walking is the best form of aerobic exercise! Why? – it brings most of the body into action which helps open up blocked blood vessels and builds your endurance. Your heart grows in strength and efficiency,

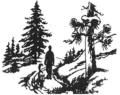

able to function with less strain! Also, many problems and upsets get solved on walks. As you walk, grasp yourself in the small of back, then press knuckles into back pains for 3 minute sessions. Your entire frame responds to every step. Feel how chief muscles function rhythmically. No other exercise gives the same harmony of coordinating sinews and same perfect circulation of blood. Brisk power walking is ideal for you, your health and your heart!

Walk 2 to 3 Miles Daily – It Does Miracles! Get Fit – Firm Up – Lose Fat – De-Stress

You should try to walk 2-3 miles daily, and some times try doubling it. *Make a daily walk a permanent part of your Bragg Healthy Heart Fitness Program* – all year and in all climates. Conrad Hilton walked in the sun and rain and loved it (page 201). Regardless of what other exercises you do, your daily walk is a *must*! Walking is what your heart needs. We are inclined to agree with Mark Twain, who said, *Golf is a good way to spoil a good walk.* But, if it takes the game to make you walk, do so. The result is almost the same – healthy functioning muscles and quickened blood circulation, plus a sense of harmony and happiness!

Although the outdoors is preferable where you can get the most fresh air – indoor walking is far better than none at all. In winter, you can try hallways, porches or shopping malls. When on our Bragg Health Crusades around the world, we enjoyed evening brisk walks through corridors, and up and down stairs of our hotel.

Expert Advice on How to Exercise

Often you may ask yourself, *"Why am I not closing in on my ideal weight?"* You're trying to workout and exercise, but your bathroom scale isn't showing you any results – your weight appears the same as when you started out. Here are some tips from the exercise experts:

Take a short walk after a meal! Taking a 15 minute stroll soon after you eat keeps blood sugar levels low and steady for the next three hours. The movement encourages muscles to use more sugar from your bloodstream.

- An effective weekly exercise program to get your heart in shape should include one rigorous program that makes you sweat; two moderate exercise programs, and one easy session. For example: taking an aerobics class, or a run and after a more relaxing yoga or stretching class.

- Daily drink 8 glasses of distilled water. This has a huge effect on exercise. Dehydrated exercisers worked out 25% less than those who drank water before, during and after exercise.

- In the initial phases of exercise training, you may get a post-workout drop in blood sugar that causes cravings for simple carbohydrates like sweets. However, cravings should disappear a few weeks into your exercise training. Have delicious fresh fruits handy such as organic apples, oranges, pears and bananas, rather than reaching for an unhealthy candy bar or soft drink filled with sugar.

To Enjoy Your Daily Walk Is Important

Your walking should never be done self-consciously. Let it be the most functional and enjoyable of exercises. Walk naturally – with head high, spine stretched up, chest out, tummy in. Swing hips, arms and body into action. Walk as though legs begin at the middle of torso. Breathe deeply! You will feel physical elation and will carry yourself proudly with body erect and arms swinging easily from shoulders. Move at your own pace, with a free spirit and a light heart. If you want, listen to motivational podcasts or music. As you walk, your body ceases to matter, you become as near a poet and nature philosopher as you will ever be.

Walk your worries away! As blood courses through your arteries and veins, cleansing and nourishing your body, you are filled with a sense of well-being that clears your mind of troubles and nourishes it with healthy positive thoughts. **When on walks and hikes Dad and I enjoyed saying to ourselves and sometimes aloud with each step – *Health! Strength! Youth! Vitality! Love! for Eternity!***

You can dramatically lower your risk of dying prematurely simply by walking briskly and engaging in other aerobic activities on a regular basis. You will help to lower blood pressure and blood cholesterol, control your weight, improve your quality of life and get better quality sleep.

It's beneficial to also take a hiking tour once a year. Select interesting areas which you, your family and friends would like to see, and hike about 15 miles daily. You will broaden your knowledge of our beautiful planet and of Mother Nature, as well as help to build a more powerful, healthy and long-lasting heart.

Walking – Running – Perfect Conditioners

We love jogging and walking – because a *run a day helps keep heart attacks away!* We also have enjoyed light jogging, as practiced by athletes in training workouts. Do this with an easy sustained pace, head up, shoulders back, arms swinging naturally. All athletes and trainers worldwide consider running and jogging as perfect conditioners.

Enjoy Exercise and Jogs for Longer Life

On our world Bragg Health Crusades the first question we would ask the hotel manager was, *"Where is the nearest park where we can take our daily exercise?"* And off we would go sometime during the day. We preferred to go early in the morning or late in the afternoon. Each person, however, should choose the time best suited and available to them.

We are so pleased to find that all over the world today running and jogging are an accepted method of achieving Heart Fitness by people of all age groups. Many cities have hiking and jogging clubs, which anyone may

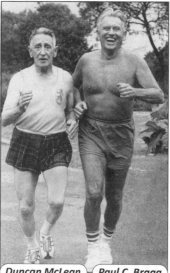

join. We have had the pleasure of running with folks everywhere we went: including Europe, England, Australia, New Zealand, Asia and throughout the U.S.

It is universally accepted that exercise is important for the promotion of physical, mental and emotional health. A daily run, jog or fast walk – when adapted

Duncan McLean   Paul C. Bragg

Paul Bragg with friend Duncan McLean, England's oldest Champion Sprinter, (83 years young) on a training run in London's beautiful Regent's Park.

to your physical and mental condition and age – will strongly improve endurance, produce a sense of well-being and help maintain total body fitness (plus each step gives your trillions of cells a massage as trampolining does also). Exercise helps increase resistance to sickness and disease, and helps make the heart healthier, fit, stronger and last longer!

Before starting your exercise program, it's wise to seek advice from your health practitioner. Also, be sure you choose a soft surface to run or jog on, such as grass or sand. Jogging on hard surfaces, such as concrete and asphalt, could accumulate damage to knees, hips, ankles and organs.

Exercise is the Best Fitness Conditioner

A daily program of walking, running or jogging is a quick, sure and inexpensive fitness conditioner. Be faithful to your exercise routine for true heart fitness. Women will be especially pleased when they see inches fly off their waistlines and hiplines – all the while improving their health! Men and women, both please remember your waistline is your lifeline and also your dateline! (see pages 67-68)

(see pages 67-68)

If you cannot get outside for your run or jog on cold and rainy days – stationary inside jogging to music or your favorite show will work too. Stay in one place and lift one foot at a time about 6-8 inches from floor – it's best to start easy and gradually build up to faster, longer periods. Enjoy exercise where you get the most fresh air – on the patio, front porch, or inside or outside rest areas at work.

Study Shows Being Fit Saves You Money

Back in 2005 the average American spent $6,683 yearly on health care. By 2020, costs almost doubled. The Centers for Disease Control (CDC) reported (back in 2000) that obesity cost the U.S. an estimated $117 billion. It is estimated direct medical costs related to physical inactivity are in the hundreds of billions as well. A study done by Dr. Tedd Mitchell of The Cooper Clinic in Dallas, Texas monitored 6,679 men. Results showed those who exercised more, required fewer doctor visits.

The Miracle Life of Jack LaLanne

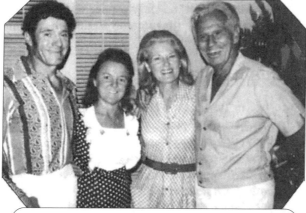

Jack, Patricia, Elaine LaLanne and Paul

Jack says he would have been dead by 17 if he hadn't attended The Bragg Crusade. Jack says, *Bragg saved my life at 15, when I attended the Bragg Health Crusade in Oakland, California.* From that day, Jack faithfully continued to live The Bragg Healthy Lifestyle, inspiring millions to health, fitness and a long and happy life! *JackLaLanne.com*

95

Being fit can cut yearly medical expenses by 25 to 60%. This study also found all you need to stay fit is to exercise just 20-30 minutes a day, 4 or 5 days a week. Physically fit people live longer and enjoy a better quality of life!

Good Shoes and Socks Promote Happy Feet

Comfortable walking shoes with flexible rubber soles under the heels is important. Insert foam inner soles, Dr. Scholl's® (*DrScholls.com*) – our friend and follower said our Bragg Foot Book is *"Best Foot Program Ever!"* Safeguard your precious feet with good serviceable shoes with ample padding! Otherwise, continual hard jarring of walking, jogging and exercising in ill-fitting or thin-soled shoes can eventually cause foot discomfort and discouragement! Shoes should not be too loose or overly tight. Feet often swell from added stimulation and circulation caused by running and when shoes are

Only 20% of American's have some form of regular exercise! This is causing poor health and more cardiovascular disease! Regular exercise is important for your Bragg Healthy Heart Program. Please start an exercise program today.

too tight you can get painful blisters! Your socks must fit right. Make sure they don't have any holes that could cause chafing or blistering. Be sure your socks aren't the kind that bunch up inside your shoes. For sports we often wear 2 pairs of socks – first a thin cotton pair, then a heavier wool – just as many tennis champs do.

Try and *do your jogging on grass, sand or soft surfaces.* Grass is easier on legs and feet, especially if you are a big person. Your legs carry you throughout life and deserve every consideration you can give them! In addition to comfortable clothes, shoes and a good exercise space, you will need willpower and a dedicated purpose to keep at it! When first starting you might be hindered by some unaccustomed aches and pains. Remember, this soreness is often a healthy sign that important fitness improvements are underway in your body. Think of any temporary discomfort in this way and you'll even take pride in feeling stiff for a few days. Take a hot apple cider vinegar bath (add 1/2 cup apple cider vinegar). The exercise rule to follow is: *train, but don't overdo and strain!*

Alternate Running and Walking
"One step begins a ten thousand mile journey."

. . . is a wise Chinese proverb to start your new, exciting journey towards Healthy Heart Fitness with a winning attitude! One yard is approximately the longest step you can take. Now, step off 25 yards or 50, 75 or 100 and slowly increase the distance and do more sets. Initially run any of these distances. If you have not been exercising, make your first weeks' daily runs 25-50 yards. Run or jog whatever distance you choose as a starter. After the run, then walk the same distance, briskly and breathing deeply while keeping your head and shoulders up and your arms swinging. Deep breathing is important. The reason you are doing this exercise is to give your heart more oxygen. Walking/running every day helps your heart get stronger!

Daily Walk and Run Brings Miracles

When you walk and run daily, the sustained pressure on the circulatory system adds elasticity to the blood vessels, increasing their capacity for greater and easier blood flow. It's remarkable that this simple exercise can be such a positive step in protecting your heart and health. A great Heart Specialist in London told us that any person who runs 15-30 minutes daily for a year could expect to double the capacity of their main arteries. *This is the way to build a powerful heart.* Activity (brisk walking, jogging, running, etc.) that causes deep breathing requires more energy! The body produces this energy by burning foodstuffs – the burning agent is oxygen. The body can store food at each meal, using what it wants and saving the rest for later, but it can't store oxygen! Most of us produce enough energy to perform ordinary daily activities. But as physical activity becomes more vigorous, the unfit just can't keep up, because the means for oxygen delivery is limited in their bodies. This is what separates the fit from the unfit!

Like a car, regular maintenance and sensible use can keep the human miracle heart working in an *as new* condition even at a vintage age! – Paul C. Bragg, N.D., Ph.D.

Jogging and running demands you to breathe more oxygen in and forces your body to process and deliver it. Even if you have been inactive or sick, start simple walking and light exercise and soon you will build better circulation, better health and increase your oxygen intake. A sound heart, like a sound car, can be driven far and fast without harm, but periods of rest and recovery are required! As we live longer, the need for rest generally increases, but not as much as most people imagine. A daily 30 minute nap is an ideal recharger after lunch.

Exercise Gives Huge Benefits for the Prevention of Heart Disease and Helps:

1. Tone muscles
2. Improve circulation
3. Lower cholesterol
4. Chase depression
5. Ease stress
6. Stimulate internal organs
7. Improve sex
8. Promote sound sleep
9. Help you think better
10. Promote deep breathing

Though no one can go back to the past and make a brand new start, you can start from right now and make a brand new healthier future!
– Carl Bard, Scottish Theologian

Importance of Abdominal (Core) Exercises

We believe that the most important exercises are those that stimulate all of the muscles of the human trunk from the hips to the armpits. These are the binding muscles which hold all of the vital organs in place. When you develop your torso's muscles, you are also developing your internal muscles and posture! As your back, waist, chest and abdomen increase in strength and elasticity, so will your lungs, heart, stomach, kidneys, etc. gain in health and efficiency. Be faithful with core exercising!

The widened arch of your ribs will give free play to your lungs. Your elastic diaphragm will allow your miracle heart to pump powerfully. Your rubber-like waist will, in its limber action, stimulate your kidneys and massage your liver. Your abdominal muscles will strengthen and support your stomach with controlled undulations. All of this strong, clean development of your torso will stimulate and help maintain the sound walls of your house and fortify the interior to resist the ravages of time. Core exercise acts like a massage of the vital organs, for that reason alone, it has a positive influence over the whole body that cannot be underestimated.

98

Now Get Started – Your Life is Precious

Start this very minute on your Heart Fitness Program! Get it firmly in your mind that you're going to build a fit heart! Banish all negative thoughts! Have faith . . . for you are now going to work with a powerful force – Mother Nature and God. Say to yourself day after day, **I am building a healthy, strong, fit heart.** Think strength and vitality for your heart. Take command of your body and mind today and let nothing distract you from faithfully following your Heart Fitness Program!

If you feel yourself weakening in your resolve, look to a Higher Power for courage and willpower! You were given one heart, one body, one life by your Creator . . . and you were given Mother Nature as your ally to help you achieve a long, healthy, fulfilled life. But no one – not even God or Mother Nature – can make you help yourself, you must do it – so now get started!

Chapter 13

Exercises For Heart Health and Good Circulation

Good Circulation – Key to a Strong Heart

When any part of the circulatory system is seriously impaired, the billions of body cells it serves are deprived of their oxygen and nourishment. With their blood supply cut off, these cells will automatically break down. The cell damage may occur in the heart itself and in the brain, the lungs, kidneys, skin or other parts of the body. Remember – if you don't use your body, you will lose it!

Five Exercises for Increased Circulation

Exercise 1 – Windmill Exercise For Energy

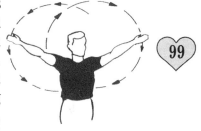

(A) Stand erect with heels and toes together, chest up, stomach drawn in, shoulders back, head high, with hands hanging loosely at your sides. Now, start swinging your arms in a forward circular motion then coming down along the sides of your body, continuing circles. Increase speed until you are making circles as fast as possible. Start by doing 10 circles forward and increase by several a day until you can bring it up to 20-30 circles at one time.

99

(B) Same position as above, only instead of making circles with the arms forward, make circles backward – in opposite direction. Start with 10 and increase to 20-30.

Exercise 2 – Hands & Finger Circulation Exercise

Stand erect as in Exercise #1. Bring hands 10 inches in front of body at chest height, and from the wrists shake the relaxed hands vigorously. Do 15 shakes with both hands at the same time and then grip hands together 15 times. Now 15 times grip each hand individually into a tight fist, then relax the hands, stretching fingers out as far as possible.

Each day is God's gift to you. Make it blossom and grow into a thing of beauty.

Exercise 3 – Body Circulation Builder

This exercise is great for people in cold climates to bring circulation to their arms, hands and upper body. Start in the same position as Exercise #1. Hold arms and hands outstretched horizontally at shoulder height. Each hand forms a half circle as the exercise is done. The right hand strikes the left shoulder and the left hand strikes the right shoulder at the same time. The arms are crisscrossed alternately with each repetition . . . right over left and then left over right. Slap the shoulders vigorously. Make it vigorous so each time the arms are flung open back to the starting position, then the chest is pushed forward and up. Start this exercise by doing 10 times and work up until you can do it 20-30 times.

Exercise 4 – Leg and Feet Vibrating Exercise

Stand erect, feet about 8-10 inches apart and arms at sides. Now, put all your weight on your left foot and raise your right foot off the ground about 6 or 8 inches. Make short stretching kicks in a forward direction. (You may hold on to a chair.) You will feel vibration from hips to toes. Now alternate, standing on right foot and kicking with your left foot. Start with 10 kicks on each foot and increase amount every day until you can kick to 20-30 times or more with each foot. Make this a vigorous exercise – it promotes great circulation to your hips, thighs, calves and feet.

Exercise 5 –Exercise for Blood Circulation in Head

Stand erect with knees relaxed and feet 12 inches apart. Lean forward from waist, with arms hanging down, relaxed near floor. (Hold on to chair if necessary.) In this position gently roll your head side to side and down and up. Do this exercise a few times in beginning, until your neck and head become accustomed to more circulation.

These simple 5 exercises cause no heart strain and are ideal for improving circulation. They help open up blocked arteries and blood vessels. When circulation is increased through exercise it helps purify the blood so more vital oxygen is carried to all parts of the body.

Exercise to Benefit the Liver and Kidneys

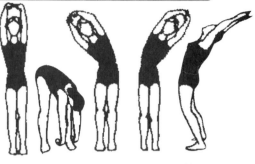

Your great filters – the kidneys – are the body's hardest working organs! Exercises that bend and twist the body at its middle will help to stimulate the kidneys, which helps them function more efficiently.

Here's great exercise for stimulating the kidneys:

Stand up straight with hands over head. Now bend forward from waist with knees relaxed and try to touch toes. Return your hands overhead, now bend backwards as far as comfortable. Now, arms up, hands clasped, bend first to left side, then to right side as far as possible. Since most of the body's liquid waste is eliminated through the kidneys, you should do these kidney stimulating exercises daily. Start with 10 of each and work up to 30.

Exercises – Good For Heart, Nerves & Health

A normal, healthy heart cannot be injured by these exercises. Start slowly and work up to a vigorous workout. Just as exercise is good for any muscle, these circulatory exercises are beneficial for both a healthy and an injured heart. These exercises will condition your heart just as they do your visible muscles. Refuse to listen to people who try to frighten you away from exercise! The heart is a muscular organ and must be exercised if it is to remain strong. By exercising you will build a stronger heart and body!

Do these exercises daily – in only 15 minutes. This is just a little time to invest in a healthy heart and a healthful life! If you have a sedentary job, if you spend a lot of time sitting or standing, do these exercises 2 or 3 times daily. When on long automobile drives, stop and do exercises every few hours. The more you do these exercises, the healthier and better circulation your body will enjoy.

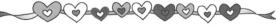

Nervous Tension can ruin your health in dozens of ways, diminish your productivity and even shorten your lifespan. – Dr. E. Jacobson, "You Must Relax"

The Dangers of Sitting too Long

Although most waste products are eliminated through the kidneys and colon, the lungs expel carbon dioxide. In the lungs tiny alveoli, blood discharges carbon dioxide and takes on oxygen, again turning bright red. It then flows back into heart, to be pumped out through the arteries to the rest of the body. This powerful cycle is repeated thousands of times daily. This is why you must never sit too long at one time. *Sitting slows down the circulation and stagnates the blood. Long periods of sitting can be damaging to the heart.* And please, never cross your legs – it's unhealthy!

People who sit for too long may develop a thrombosis (blood clot) in the deep veins of the calf. If your office

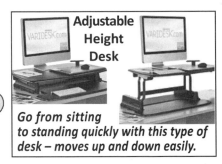

Adjustable Height Desk

Go from sitting to standing quickly with this type of desk – moves up and down easily.

work requires sitting a lot, *get up, move around every hour or get an adjustable height desk.* On long car trips, stop every two hours and take a walk or do exercises. When exercising, you flush out toxins and stimulate vital blood circulation.

The Art of Healthy Sitting

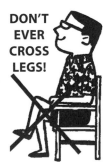

DON'T EVER CROSS LEGS!

When sitting, please sit correctly! *The most disastrous and injurious habit of bad sitting is crossing the legs* for it compresses the popliteal artery in the back of the knees which can cause a variety of unhealthy problems (blood stagnation in the hips, legs, knees, and feet plus backaches, varicose veins, hemorrhoids, headaches, and pain).

When you sit in a chair, sit well back. Do not let the edge of the chair cut off circulation in the back of the knees. Keep your feet on floor. Dangling your legs puts too much pressure on veins. Adults who have shorter legs should use a box or footstool. We love rocking chairs – you get rest by sitting, plus peaceful (helps solve problems) rocking exercise!

Exercise (Sweating) is Healthy for You!

The skin, with its millions of pores and sweat glands, is the body's largest eliminating organ – (often called the third kidney). Sweat has a dual purpose – it rids the body of impurities and serves as a temperature regulator! When our body is exposed to heat or *warmed up* by exercise, sweat glands are stimulated into action. Evaporation of the sweat cools the blood when it reaches the skin. This helps the body from becoming overheated and, at the same time, eliminates impurities near the skin's surface.

It's the toxic impurities or the mixture with skin dirt, that gives sweat a bad odor. If you are clean inside and out, then there is only the good sweat smell. Regardless of what deodorant advertisers say, *it's healthy to sweat.* From dancing, calisthenics, walking, cycling and even vigorous housework, to saunas and steam rooms – any activity that makes you sweat improves your heart action and health. Hard work never hurts when you're healthy!

Indulge in Hobbies that are Active and Fun

We promote Healthy Heart crusading against inactivity, long sitting and sedentary activities that slow down body circulation. When that happens changes take place in the artery walls! You must keep active! Cultivate fun hobbies that give needed exercise you can enjoy, such as hiking, swimming, tennis, dancing, gardening, golf, etc. You can't build a strong heart unless you exercise, walk briskly, bend, twist, and use your muscles which promotes healthy overall body circulation! Remember stagnation breeds disease.

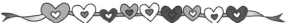

You have to eat healthy and exercise to treat your arteries and heart well. If you don't challenge your body by working it through exercise, brisk walking, etc. your heart muscle and entire cardiovascular system will not work at their best!

It's a lean, fit horse for the long, healthy successful race of life! – Paul C. Bragg

Massages help increase blood circulation, lower levels of stress hormones, and reduces heart rate and blood pressure. To prevent frequent tension headaches, consider getting massages. Migraine sufferers who receive regular massages have fewer attacks, need less medication and sleep better. – Dr. Andrew Weil

Avoid Constricting Clothes and Shoes

Anything that impedes blood circulation damages the heart and its arterial and vascular systems. Therefore, wear no constricting undergarments – this includes tight bras,* belts, collars, ties and above all, tight shoes.

Tight shoes can do more to disturb the circulation than any other article of clothing because the feet must always be well supplied with blood. There are 26 bones in each foot – more than any other part of the body. When blood does not reach the feet in required quantities, toxins are retained in the feet cells. That is why so many people's feet have unpleasant odors – they need to cleanse their body!

Many unhealthy conditions of stiffness, deformities and pain are brought on by ill-fitting shoes that cause poor circulation and incorrect posture when walking and standing! Only wear comfortable, practical shoes that don't bind or inhibit the free blood circulation in the feet.

Exercise & Earthing Builds Better Circulation

Walking barefoot is the ideal way to walk. Each time we remove our shoes and walk barefoot is an opportunity to improve our circulation! Walking or light jogging on grass, sand, bare soil or simply walking barefoot around the house improves circulation with each step and helps strengthen the heart! When our bare feet come into contact with Earth (known as Earthing), it gives us a charge of energy which helps to restore a natural electrical balance in our body.

The heart must pump blood to the legs and feet, as well as to the arms and hands. Most people do not have sufficient rhythmic circulation to these extremities. That is why so many people complain of cold feet and legs that *go to sleep* easily and arms and hands that become cold and numb. Next page is a hydro-therapeutic water therapy that helps alleviate these conditions.

For more info on "Earthing" check out these websites:
● *www.Earthing.com* ● *www.EarthingInstitute.net*

*Please read "Dressed to Kill" by Sydney Singer on breast cancer and bra studies.
(I prefer not to wear a bra but instead a loose chemise. - Patricia Bragg)

Cold and Hot Water Circulation Therapy**

Get two foot tubs or wash tubs. Fill one with hot water – about 104° or as hot as desired. Fill the other with cold water, preferably with ice cubes added. Now for 2 minutes put your feet in hot water and entire lower arms (hands to elbows) submerged in cold water. After 2 minutes reverse the procedure – put feet in cold water, arms and hands in hot water for another 2 minutes. Repeat this cycle five times, then take a coarse cotton towel and rub your feet, arms and hands vigorously until they are warm and glowing with tingling, healthy circulation!

Here's another healthy water therapy to stimulate foot circulation. Sit on chair next to bathtub with your feet dangling over tub; turn on strong flow of water and for 5-10 minutes, alternate hot and cold water over your feet. Finish up with a massage and coarse towel rub.

Shower Therapy Builds Healthy Circulation

Here's a progressive method for improving circulation over your entire body. All you need is a large back brush or Swedish bath friction mitt, Castile soap and a coarse Turkish towel. Get into shower and turn on mild hot water. With brush or mitt, gently scrub your body. At first your coddled body won't be able to take too much scrubbing. Also give a good hand-massage to your body, neck and shoulders. After scrub/massage part, alternate hot and cold showers every 2 to 3 minutes.* Now towel rub your body dry for 3 to 5 minutes – your circulation will tingle!

It's wonderful relaxation for tired or sore muscles and a refreshing stimulation with a hot/cold water shower* letting spray beat heavily on back and shoulders. Twice weekly, before showering massage oil onto skin. We advise this relaxing shower before dinner on days when you come home tired. It refreshes and relaxes you!

**Alternating hot and cold water treatments will stimulate circulation and helps strengthen the body's immune system. – Father Sebastian Kneipp, German Pioneer in Holistic Healing and Father of Hydrotherapy. – Kneipp.com

---

*Use a filtered shower head to remove chlorine, lead, mercury, arsenic, iron, hydrogen sulfide, bacteria, fungi, dirt and sediment from your water. I have been using a shower filter for years and enjoy my chlorine-free showers!
– Patricia Bragg

Great Framingham 50 Year Heart Study

In 1948 in Framingham, MA, 2,336 men and 2,873 women participated in a landmark study, *The Framingham Heart Study*. This ongoing study is still the source of much of our present understanding of heart disease and stroke. The original study group of 1948 and the succeeding generation of Framingham residents have been followed throughout their lives. Everyone has been interviewed every two years for over 70 years. This massive pioneer medical research has been renewed and continues on today.

In 1971, the original Framingham subjects were joined by 5,135 of their children. The researchers were pleased to find a 43% reduction in heart disease deaths from the 1948 group. *The New England Journal of Medicine* says the increasing heart-health of Framingham's 1970's test group is primarily results of their lifestyle improvements. They reduced cholesterol, lowered blood pressure and abstained from unhealthy foods and smoking factors that so harmed the early 1950's group.

Dr. T. Colin Campbell's China Project

In another landmark study, the *China Project*, written by Dr. T. Colin Campbell, the effects of nearly 50 disease categories on counties in the US and China were observed for 20 years. Results showed that populations using a diet richer in animal products and higher in total fat were much more afflicted with chronic degenerative diseases (cancers, cardiovascular diseases, diabetes, etc.). The Chinese diet contains 0 to 20% animal-based foods, while the affluent rich American diet, sad to say, is comprised of 50 to 70%. What's worse, far more Americans are clinically obese, even though the Chinese consume 30% more total calories! Another astonishing fact is that China's high cholesterol levels are almost equal to the U.S.'s low!

I live on legumes, vegetables and fruits. No dairy, no meat of any kind – no chicken, no turkey, very little fish, once in a while. It changed my metabolism and I lost 24 pounds. I did research and found 82% of people who go on a plant-based diet begin to heal themselves, as I did. – U.S. President Bill Clinton, 1993-2001

When you increase strength training, brisk walking becomes easier and lets you walk faster and farther, which gives the heart and lungs a better workout.

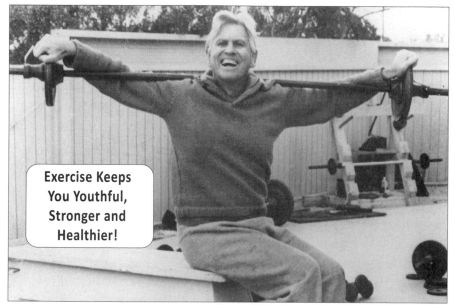

Exercise Keeps
You Youthful,
Stronger and
Healthier!

Paul C. Bragg and Patricia enjoyed lifting weights 3 times weekly.

What these two ambitious studies have to say about maintaining cardiovascular health is just what we've been telling people for years! Eat a natural diet low in fats, cholesterol, sugars, salts, etc.; exercise regularly; fast; don't smoke – this is *The Bragg Healthy Lifestyle!*

Landmark U.S. Government Study Iron-Pumping Oldsters (ages 86-96) Triple Muscle Strength in 1990

WASHINGTON, June 13, 1990 – Ageing nursing home residents in Boston *pumping iron?* Elderly weight-lifters tripling and quadrupling muscle strength? Is it possible? Most people would wonder at this amazing revelation!

Yet U.S. Government Experts on ageing answered those questions with a resounding *"YES"* according to results of study. They turned a group of frail Boston nursing home residents, aged 86 to 96, into weight-lifters to demonstrate that it's never too late to reverse age-related declines in muscle strength! The study group participated in a regime of high-intensity weight-training in research conducted by Agriculture Departments Human Research Center of Ageing at Tufts University in Boston. *A high-intensity weight training program is capable of inducing dramatic increases in muscle strength in frail men and women up to 96 years of age,* reported by the study director, Dr. Maria A. Fiatarone.

Amazing Health & Fitness Results in 8 Weeks

Despite their many handicaps, the elderly weightlifters increased their muscle strength by 3-4 times as much in as little as 8 weeks. Dr. Fiatarone said they probably were stronger at the end of the program than they had been in years!

Dr. Fiatarone and her associates emphasized the safety of such a closely supervised weight-lifting program, even among people in frail health. The average age of the ten participants was 90. Six had coronary heart disease, seven had arthritis, six had bone fractures resulting from osteoporosis, four had high blood pressure, and all had been physically inactive for years. Yet no serious medical problems resulted from this program. A few of the participants did report minor muscle and joint aches, but 9 of the 10 still completed the program. One man, aged 86, felt a pulling sensation at the site of a previous hernia incision and dropped out after four weeks.

The study participants were drawn from a 712-bed long-term care facility in Boston, Massachusetts and worked out three times a week during this study. They performed three sets of 8 repetitions with each leg on a weight lifting machine. The weights were gradually increased from 10 lbs. to 40 lbs. at the end of the 8 week program.

Muscle strength in the average adult decreases by 30% to 50% during the course of a lifetime. Muscle atrophy and weakness is not merely a cosmetic problem in elderly people, but especially frail elderly. Researchers have linked muscle weakness with recurrent falls, which is a major cause of immobility and death with the American elderly! This is costing the U.S. billions of dollars yearly in staggering medical fees.

Previous studies have suggested that weight training can be helpful in reversing age-related muscle weakness. But Dr. Fiatarone said physicians have been reluctant to recommend weight lifting for frail elderly patients with multiple health problems. This 1990 government study should help change their minds. **The study shows the importance of keeping the 640 body muscles as active and fit as possible to maintain good physical fitness, plus good heart and body health!**

Chapter 14

Doctor Pure Water

Pure Water Helps Keep Body Clean Inside

To have a clean, healthy bloodstream and arteries free of corrosion, we must not only eat correctly, but also drink the right fluids. ***The liquids which go into our bodies must be pure, nourishing and healthy.*** To begin with, we believe every person should have the equivalent of *8-10 glasses purified or distilled water daily.* It can be obtained in most supermarkets, grocery stores and health stores. Or look for local bottled water suppliers or you can buy a water distiller machine.

Distilled water has no inorganic minerals to deposit on the artery walls and other *pipes* of the body. In contrast, most sources of *well, spring and river waters all contain inorganic minerals and some even have toxic chemicals which cannot ever be utilized in the body chemistry.* They can corrode the human *pipes* just as they do the plumbing pipes which bring water into your home.

109

Hard Water Causes Hard Arteries

The human body has a vast piping system called the bloodstream. A healthy heart must have clean, open coronary arteries. The blood must be able to flow through them smoothly to nourish the heart and keep it pumping steadily and efficiently (it is our miracle muscle pump).

Suppose a person drinks only the hard chemicalized water and their pipelines become clogged and blocked by the inorganic minerals which can not be absorbed into the body. Blockage in the coronary arteries feeding the heart, reduces the amount of blood reaching the heart. When the blood supply is reduced enough, the affected parts of the heart cease to function. A heart attack and even death may result when some sections of the heart muscle stop functioning.

Distilled water plays a vital part in the treatment of illness, arthritis, etc.
– Dr. Banik

The Difference Between Organic and Inorganic Minerals

Inorganic minerals never lived and are inert . . . which means that they *cannot be absorbed into the body!*

Organic minerals are those which come from that which is *living* or has lived . . . and *16 of these organic minerals are essential elements of the human body.* When we eat an apple or any other fruit or vegetable, that substance is living, for it has a certain lifespan after it has been picked. The same is true of animal foods, such as fish, milk, cheese and eggs. Animals obtain their organic minerals from plants. We humans obtain our organic minerals from both plants and animals.

Only a living plant has the power to extract inorganic minerals from the earth and sun and change them into organic minerals. No animal or human can do this. If you were stranded on an uninhabited island where nothing was growing, you would starve to death. Although the soil beneath your feet would contain all 16 *essential* minerals, your body could not absorb them.

110

Organic Minerals are vital in keeping us alive and healthy, but Inorganic Minerals can stiffen, sicken and can slowly kill us!

Pure water is the best drink for a wise man. – Henry David Thoreau

Most Americans' bodies thirst for pure distilled water! Their bodies can become sick, prematurely aged, crippled and stiff due to inorganic minerals, chemicalized water and lack of sufficient pure water!

WATER IS KEY TO HEALTH & ALL BODY FUNCTIONS:

- Heart
- Circulation
- Digestion
- Bones & Joints
- Muscles
- Metabolism
- Assimilation
- Elimination
- Nerves
- Energy
- Sex
- Glands

Water flows through every single part of your body, cleansing and nourishing it. But the wrong kind of water, with inorganic minerals, harmful toxins, chemicals and other contaminants can pollute and clog your body, gradually stiffening it painfully. – Paul C. Bragg, N.D., Ph.D.

Hard Water is Unhealthy

For years we've heard people claim that certain waters were rich in all the minerals. What minerals are they talking about? Inorganic or organic? If they are inorganic, people are simply burdening their bodies with inert minerals which may cause the development of stones in the kidneys and the gallbladder and acid crystals in the arteries, veins, joints and other parts of the body.

Vegetable and Fruit Juices Contain Mother Nature's Distilled Water

No new water has been put on the face of Mother Earth since it was originally formed. Just as the same energy is formed and re-formed, so the same water is used and re-used over and over again by the miracle of Mother Nature. Waters of the earth are purified by distillation. The sun evaporates the water which is collected into clouds. When the clouds become full we have rain and dew – pure, perfectly clean, distilled water, free of all harmful inorganic substances, until polluted!

Years ago, when the late actor Douglas Fairbanks Sr. and Dad were close friends, they roamed the South Sea Islands for several months. During that trip Dad came upon an island inhabited by *beautiful, healthy Polynesians* who drank only distilled water because the island was surrounded by the Pacific Ocean. Their island was based on porous coral which could not hold water – so they

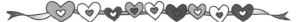

Water from chemically treated public water systems – and even from many wells and springs – is likely to be loaded with poisonous chemicals and toxic trace elements. Depending upon the kinds of pipes used in the buildings, the water is likely to be overloaded with lead (from older, soldered pipe joints), zinc (from old-fashioned galvanized pipes) or with copper and cadmium (from copper pipes). These trace elements are released in dangerous quantities by the chemical action of the water flowing against the metals of the pipes.

Water flows throughout your body, cleansing and nourishing it. But the wrong kind of water – with inorganic minerals, harmful toxins and contaminants, can clog and gradually turn your body into stone.

would *only drink rain water* or the fresh, clear, clean water of the green coconut. Dad had never seen any finer specimens of humanity than these native South Sea Islanders. There were several doctors on the yacht who thoroughly examined the most mature people on these islands. One heart doctor stated that he had never in his life examined such healthy, well-preserved people.

You may have noted we said only the most mature people were examined by the doctors. *They were so completely unaware of age* that no such word existed in their language! They never celebrated birthdays, so they were forever young – gloriously ageless, not only in years, but in body! These older men performed as well in the vigorous native dances, as the younger men. They were all beautiful human specimens because they lived their lengthy lives drinking only pure distilled water, eating natural foods and enjoying an active, healthy lifestyle.

Why We Drink Only Distilled Water

Sadly, in some areas it's no longer safe to drink rain or snow water because of man's vast reach of polluting the air! But when you drink fresh juices of organic fruits and vegetables, remember all of this liquid has been *distilled by Mother Nature* and is 100% inorganic mineral-free. Organic fruit and vegetable juices contain Mother Nature's pure distilled water, plus important nutrients such as natural sugars, organic minerals and vitamins.

You will hear people say, *distilled water is dead water, a fish cannot live in it.* Of course fish cannot live in distilled water for any length of time! They need the vegetation that grows in rivers, lakes and seas to live.

Another erroneous distilled water notion is that it *leaches the organic minerals out of the body*. This is 100% false! It leaches out inorganic minerals, which you want to be rid of that can cause you painful health problems.

It's excellent for detoxification – *distilled water helps to dissolve and flush out the terrible toxic poisons that collect in our bodies.* This pure water helps to eliminate these toxic poisons through the kidneys without painful buildup that the inorganic crystals and the stones create.

Distilled Water is World's Purest, Best Water!

Every liquid prescription that is mixed in any drug store the world over is prepared with distilled water. It is used in baby formulas and for many hundreds of other purposes where absolutely pure water is essential.

Distilled water is NOT soft water. Water softeners are being used in millions of homes because hard water is not ideal for washing your hair, clothes, dishes, etc. If you wash your hair in soft water you will discover how soft it is. *But please do not drink the water out of water softeners!* It's not healthy for you to drink and cook your food with because of its salt and chemical content.

At the Bragg home we have used a water distiller and for our office staff we have distilled water delivered in 5 gallon bottles. Try distilled water for a year, you will see the results and never want to drink hard water again!

Pure, distilled water is vitally important in following The Bragg Healthy Lifestyle and water is key to all body functions (see page 110). The right kind of water is one of your best natural protections against all kinds of diseases and viral infections, flu, etc. It's the vital factor in all body fluids, tissues, cells, lymph, blood and all glandular secretions. Water holds all nutritive factors in solution, as well as toxins and body wastes, and acts as the main transportation medium throughout the body, for both nutritional and important cleansing purposes!

113

Drinking water at correct times maximizes body effectiveness!

- Two glasses of distilled water in the morning helps activate your internal organs.
- A glass of water before taking a bath/shower helps to lower your blood pressure.
- Drinking water 2-3 hours before bedtime, helps you avoid a stroke or heart attack.
- A glass of water with apple cider vinegar 30 minutes before meals, helps to improve digestion, gerd and glucose levels. – Gabriel Cousens, M.D.

The 75% Watery Human

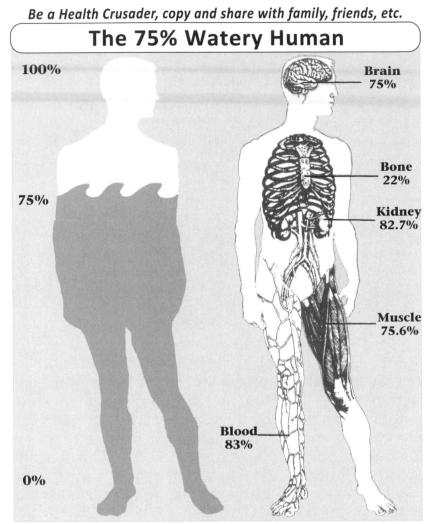

100%

75%

75%

0%

114

Brain
75%

Bone
22%

Kidney
82.7%

Muscle
75.6%

Blood
83%

The amount of water in the body, averaging 75%, varies considerably and even from one part of the body to another area (illustration on right). A lean man may hold 75% of his weight in body water, while a woman – because of her larger proportion of water-poor fatty tissues – may be only 52% water. The lowering of water content in the blood is what triggers the hypothalamus, the brain's vital thirst center, to send out its familiar urgent demand for a drink of water! Please obey and drink ample amounts of purified water. By the time you feel thirsty, you're already dehydrated.
– American Running and Fitness Association

Water Percentage in Various Body Parts:

Teeth	10%	Spleen	75.5%
Bones	22%	Lungs	80%
Cartilage	55%	Blood	83%
Red blood corpuscles	68.7%	Bile	86%
Liver	71.5%	Plasma	90%
Brain	75%	Lymph	94%
Muscle tissue	75%	Saliva	95.5%

This chart shows why 8-10 glasses of pure water daily is so important.

Ten Common Sense Reasons Why Distilled Water is Optimal!

- There are over 80,000 toxic chemicals on the market today and over 500 are being added yearly! Wherever you live, in the city or on the farm, some of these chemicals are getting into your drinking water. Beware of toxic chemicalized water.

- No one on the face of the earth today knows what effect these chemicals have on the body as they blend into thousands of different combinations. It is like making a mixture of colors; one drop could change the color.

- Proper equipment hasn't been designed yet to detect some of these chemicals, and may not be for years to come.

- The miracle working body is made up of 75% water. Therefore, don't you think you should be wise, particular and cautious about the type of water you put in your body?

- The Navy has been drinking distilled water for years!

- Distilled water is chemical and mineral free. Distillation removes all the chemicals and impurities from water that are possible to remove. If distillation doesn't remove them, there is no known method today that will.

- The body does need minerals . . . but it is not necessary that they come from water. There is not one mineral in water which cannot be found more abundantly in food! Water is the most unreliable source of minerals because it varies from one area to another. The healthy food we eat – is the best source of organic minerals, not the water we drink!

- Distilled water is used for intravenous feeding, inhalation therapy, prescriptions and baby formulas. Therefore, doesn't it make sense that distilled water is good for everyone?

- Thousands of water distillers have been sold throughout the United States and around the world to individuals, families, dentists, doctors, hospitals, nursing homes and government agencies. These informed, alert consumers are helping protect their health by using only steam distilled water. They don't want to drink the toxic, harmful chemicals.

- With chemicals, pollutants and other impurities in our water, it makes good sense to clean up the water you drink using Mother Nature's inexpensive way – distillation.

Pure distilled water is truly god's greatest gift to us – it's the vital natural chemistry of life, and a source of health. – Paul C. Bragg, N.D., Ph.D.

Pure Water is Key!

Although distilled water may be optimal, drinking pure untreated water from a credible water company, reverse osmosis unit, or a clear well will greatly improve your health and vitality. In fact, it's one of the best things you can do for yourself and your family. "Pure water" is water that has had all contaminants removed. And, whenever possible, avoid plastic bottles. Instead use glass or stainless steel.

Fluorine is a Deadly Poison!

Millions of innocent people have been brainwashed by the aluminum companies to erroneously believe that adding sodium fluoride (their waste by-product) to our drinking water will reduce tooth decay in our children. Americans get sodium fluoride in their drinking water without thinking about it. Sodium fluorine, a chemical "cousin" of sodium fluoride, is used as a rat and roach killer and a deadly pesticide! Yet this deadly sodium fluoride, injected almost by government edict into drinking water in the proportion of 1.2 parts per million (PPM), has been declared by the U.S. Public Health Service to be *safe for all human consumption. Every chemist knows that such absolute safety is not only false but is also truly unattainable and a total illusion!*

116

Keep Toxic Fluoride Out of Your Water!

Most of the water Americans drink has fluoride in it, including tap and bottled water and canned drinks and foods! The ADA (American Dental Association) is insisting that the FDA (Food and Drug Association) mandate the addition of toxic fluoride to all bottled waters! Defend your right to drink pure, non-fluoridated tap and bottled waters! Challenge and stop local and state water fluoridation policies! Call, write, fax or e-mail all your state officials and Congress people and send them a copy of this book.

CHECK FOLLOWING WEBSITES FOR FLUORIDE UPDATES:

- Fluoride.Mercola.com
- www.FluorideResearch.org
- www.FluorideAlert.org
- www.Fluoridation.com

Showers, Toxic Chemicals & Chlorine

Water chlorination has been widely used to "purify" water in this country for most of this century. But its negative effects on health surely outweigh any benefits. "Chlorine is the greatest crippler and killer of modern times. While it prevented epidemics of one disease, it was creating another. Twenty years after the start of chlorinating our drinking water in 1904, the present mounting epidemic of heart trouble, cancer and senility began and is costing billions."
– Dr. Joseph Price, *Coronaries/Cholesterol/Chlorine*

The skin absorption of toxic dangerous contaminants has been greatly underestimated and the ingestion may not constitute the sole primary route of toxic exposure.
– Dr. Halina Brown, *American Journal of Public Health*

Taking long hot showers is a health risk, according to the latest research. Showers – and to a lesser extent baths – lead to a greater exposure to toxic chemicals contained in water supplies than does drinking the water. These toxic chemicals evaporate out of the water and are inhaled. They can also spread through the house and be inhaled by others. People get six to 100 times more chemicals by breathing the air while taking showers and baths than they would by drinking the water. – Ian Anderson

A Professor of Water Chemistry at the University of Pittsburgh claims that exposure to vaporized chemicals in the water through showering, bathing and inhalation is 100 times greater than through drinking the chemicals in water.
– *Troubled Waters on Tap*

Angina, allergies, asthma, back and joint pains, migraines, stomach pains and arthritis may be symptoms of severe dehydration – which is easily helped by drinking 8-10 glasses of purified distilled water daily! Start increasing your water intake today. Be water wise and health safe! – Paul C. Bragg, N.D., Ph.D.

There is only one water that is clean and that is steam distilled water. No other substance on our planet does so much to keep us healthy and get us well as distilled water does. – Dr. James Balch, Co-Author, "Dietary Wellness"

Don't gamble with your health, use a shower filter to remove chlorine, fluoride, bacteria, toxins, etc. I have been using a water filter for years and enjoy my safe, chlorine-free showers! – Patricia Bragg

Five Hidden Toxic Dangers in Your Shower:

● **Chlorine:** Added to all municipal water supplies, this disinfectant hardens arteries, destroys proteins in the body, irritates skin and sinus conditions and aggravates any asthma, allergies and respiratory problems.

● **Chloroform:** This powerful by-product of chlorination causes excessive free radical formation (a cause of accelerated ageing! see page 26-27), normal cells to mutate and cholesterol to form. It's a known carcinogen!

● **DCA (Dichloroacetic acid):** This chlorine by-product alters cholesterol metabolism and has been shown to cause liver cancer in lab animals.

● **MX (toxic chlorinated acid):** Another by-product of chlorination, MX is known to cause genetic mutations that can lead to cancer growth and has been found in all chlorinated water for which it was tested.

● **Proven cause of bladder and rectal cancer:** Research proved that chlorinated water is the direct cause of 9% of all U.S. bladder cancers and 15% of all rectal cancers.

118

Don't Gamble With Your Health – Use a Shower Filter That Removes Toxins

The most effective method of removing hazards from your shower is the quick and easy installation of a filter on your shower arm. The best filter we found removes chlorine, fluoride, lead, mercury, iron, chlorine by-products, arsenic, hydrogen sulfide, and other unseen toxic contaminants, such as bacteria, fungi, dirt and sediments. It has a 12-18 month filter life-span and you can easily clean the filter by backwashing and replace only when needed.

Start enjoying safe, chlorine-free showers right away. It's essential to reducing your risk of heart disease and cancer and to ease the strain on your immune system. And you may even get rid of long-standing conditions – from sinus and respiratory problems to dry, itchy skin.

"Water contains healing; it is the simplest, cheapest and – if used correctly – the safest remedy. Water is my best friend and will remain all my life!"
– Father Sebastian Kneipp, Father of Hydrotherapy • www.Kneipp.com

You Get More Toxic Exposure from Taking a Chlorinated Water Shower Than From Drinking the Same Water!

Two of the very highly toxic and volatile chemicals, trichloroethylene and chloroform, have been proven as toxic contaminants found in most all municipal drinking U.S. water supplies. The National Academy of Sciences recently has estimated that hundreds of people die in the United States each year from the cancers caused largely by ingesting water pollutants from inhalation as air pollutants in the home. Inhalation exposure to water pollutants is largely ignored. Recent shocking data indicates that hot showers can liberate about 50% of the chloroform and 80% of the trichloroethylene into the air.

Tests show your body can absorb more toxic chlorine from a 10 minute shower than drinking 8 glasses of the same water. How can that be? A warm shower opens up your pores, causing your skin to act like a sponge. As a result, you not only inhale the toxic chlorine vapors, you absorb them through your skin, directly into your bloodstream – at a toxic rate that is up to 6 times higher than drinking it.

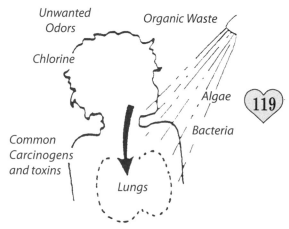

In terms of cumulative damage to your health, showering in chlorinated water is one of the most dangerous risks you take daily. Short-term risks include: eye, sinus, throat, skin and lung irritation. Long-term risks include: excessive free radical formation (that ages you!), higher vulnerability to genetic mutation and cancer development; and difficulty metabolizing cholesterol that can cause hardened arteries. – Science News

The treatment of diseases should go to the root of the cause. Often it is found in severe dehydration from lack of purified water, and an unhealthy lifestyle!

Distillation effectively removes the widest variety of toxins and contaminants from water. – David and Anne Frahm, authors of "Healthy Habits"

119

Comparison of Water Treatment Methods
Show Steam Distilled Water is the Best

Pollutant	Sediment Filter	Carbon Filter	Reverse Osmosis	Steam Distillation
Aluminum	○	○	●	●
Arsenic	○	○	◐	●
Bacteria	○	○	◐	●
Benzene	○	○	●[1]	●[1]
Bromide	○	○	●	●
Cadmium	○	○	●	●
Calcium	○	○	●	●
Chlorides	○	●	●	●
Chlorine	○	●	●[1]	●[1]
Chromium (VI)	○	◐	●[1]	●[1]
Cryptosporidium	○	○	●	●
Detergents	○	◐	●	●
Fluorides	○	○	●	●
Herbicides	○	●	●[1]	●[1]
Lead	○	○	●	●
Magnesium	○	○	●	●
Mercury	○	○	●	●
MTBE	○	●	●[1]	●[1]
Nitrate	○	○	◐	●
Organics	○	●	●[1]	●[1]
Pesticides	○	●	●[1]	●[1]
Phosphates	○	○	●	●
Radon	○	○	●[1]	●[1]
Sediment	●	◐	●	●
Sodium	○	○	●	●
Sulfates	○	◐	●	●
Sulfide	○	◐	●	●
TDS	○	○	●	●
TTHM	○	○	●[1]	●[1]
Viruses	○	○	○	●

○ *Ineffective or No Reduction*　◐ *Significant Reduction*　● *Effective Removal*

1 – A Carbon Filter Needed (The best home distillers also have carbon filters.)

120

The kind of water you drink can make or break you – your body is 75% water.

Chapter 15

Doctor Healthy Foods

Eating for Super Health and Longevity

In this "Bragg Heart Fitness Program" we have been emphasizing the *dont's* because we consider these much more difficult to follow than the *do's*. Now we will detail what kind of food program you should follow for heart fitness, health and living a longer, healthier life.

Every time you plan a meal, check off these items on the fingers of your hand to see if you are eating a *nutritionally well-balanced combination of foods: protein, carbohydrates, fats, fruits and vegetables.*

1. PROTEIN: *The Building Blocks of the Body*

Protein foods are raw nuts (walnuts, almonds), seeds (chia, flax, pumpkin, sesame, sunflower), wheat germ, beans, dairy products, whole grain cereals, meat, fish, poultry and protein supplements. Protein is one of the most important food elements and *is essential for keeping the heart fit.* You must have protein for building every cell of your body. This fundamental demand of Mother Nature rules every creature living on the face of Earth, including man.

Protein is you – flesh, muscle, blood, heart, bones, skin and hair – all the components of the body are essentially composed of protein. *You are literally "built" of protein.* This basic function of your body – of converting food into living tissue – is one of life's miracles! Your life processes and the factors that help you resist disease are all composed of protein (amino acids) components.

Every time you move a muscle, every time your heart beats, every time you breathe, you consume protein in the form of amino acids. The link between protein and body tissue is amino acids – and the bloodstream carries them to every part of the body where they work to repair, rebuild and maintain body tissues. They enrich the blood and condition the organs, including the heart.

121

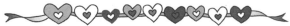

See website: www.Nutrition.gov for healthy nutritional tips!

Amino Acids – Body's Protein Building Blocks

Along with carbohydrates, fats, water, vitamins and minerals – proteins are part of the essential nutrients for the human body. Amino acids are the organic compounds that make up proteins. Specifically, a protein is made up of one or more linear chains of amino acids, each of which is called a polypeptide. There are 20 types of amino acids commonly found in proteins.

Amino acids are essential to all living organisms, acting as building blocks in: muscle, hair, nails, skin and internal organs; facilitating chemical reactions in our cells; and fighting disease. Amino acids are classified into three groups: essential, non-essential and conditional.

ESSENTIAL AMINO ACIDS: Cannot be made by the body. They must come from food. There are nine essential amino acids: Histidine, Isoleucine, Leucine, Lysine, Methionine, Phenylalanine, Threonine, Tryptophan, and Valine.

NONESSENTIAL AMINO ACIDS: Means that our bodies can produce an amino acid, even if we do not get it from the food we eat. The Nonessential amino acids include: Alanine, Arginine, Asparagine, Aspartic acid, Cysteine, Glutamic Acid, Glutamine, Glycine, Proline, Serine, and Tyrosine.

CONDITIONAL AMINO ACIDS: Are usually not essential, except in times of illness and stress. Conditional amino acids include: Arginine, Cysteine, Glutamine, Tyrosine, Glycine, Ornithine, Proline, and Serine.

You do not need to eat essential and nonessential amino acids at every meal, but getting a balance of them over the whole day is important. Just look at the adequacy of the diet overall throughout the day.

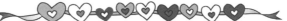

Amino acids are essential for production of energy within ourselves, for detoxification and for vital transmission of nerve impulses. In short, they are the very soup of life, and are almost always overlooked and neglected.
– H. J. Hoegerman, M.D.

Amino Acids are needed for building every part of the body: bones, blood, hair, skin, nails and glands – and are Mother Nature's and God's life-giving secret to a long life. – Paul C. Bragg, N.D., Ph.D., Originator of Health Stores

Amino Acids – Life-Givers and Life-Extenders

Amino acids and proteins have the following wide and varied roles in the human body:

• **Structure:** Proteins act as structural components in the body for example with muscles, hair, nails, skin and the internal organs (the lungs, liver, kidneys, heart and intestines).

• **Repairing:** Proteins are necessary for tissue repair and the building of new tissues.

• **Enzymes:** are the catalysts in the body, which means that they make chemical reactions go faster, but are not changed by the reaction.

• **Hormone Signaling:** Hormones are used to pass messages around the body instructing our organs and tissues how to do their job.

• **Defense:** Amino acids are used to build antibodies, the "soldiers" in our immune system, essential for fighting disease and keeping us free from illness.

When you consume protein, it is broken down in the gut to its amino acid or peptide components, before being transported in the blood to where it is needed.

How Much Protein Do We Need?

How much protein you need depends on your body weight, your body fat and your physical activity (see chart page 134).

The DRI (Dietary Reference Intake) is 0.8 grams of protein per kilogram of body weight (0.36 grams per pound). This amounts to: 56 grams per day for the average sedentary man, 46 grams per day for the average woman. This must include a balance of each of the eight essential amino acids.

If physically active, undergoing some stress or sickness, pregnant, nursing mothers, and children – add up to 30 grams a day to this basic requirement.

Each day, time is your greatest treasure, spend it wisely! – Patricia Bragg

---

Let food be your medicine, and medicine be your food. – Hippocrates, 400 B.C.

Too Much Protein in the Diet is also Detrimental to Your Health

Some weight loss programs recommend very high protein diets of up to 200 grams of proteins a day. This is way too high and can be dangerous for health! It's important to understand the health concerns related to excess protein in the body, especially if you follow an excessively high-protein diet for an extended period of time (such as the Atkins Diet).

Bad Breath: especially if you restrict your carbohydrate intake. This could be in part because your body goes into a metabolic state called ketosis, which produces chemicals that give off an unpleasant fruity smell.

Constipation: High-protein diets that restrict carbohydrates are typically low in fiber. Increasing your water and fiber intake can help prevent constipation.

Diarrhea: Eating too much dairy or processed food, coupled with a lack of fiber, can cause diarrhea.

Dehydration: Your body flushes out excess nitrogen with fluids and water. This can leave you dehydrated even though you may not feel more thirsty than usual.

Kidney damage: Protein breakdown creates side-products that give extra work to the kidneys and liver. Also a marked acid load to the kidneys can increase the risk of kidney stone formation.

Increased cancer risk: Sources have shown that certain high-protein diets that are particularly high in red meat-based protein are linked to an increased risk of various health issues, including cancer.

Heart disease: Eating lots of red meat and full-fat dairy foods as part of a high-protein diet may lead to heart disease. This could be related to higher intakes of saturated fat and cholesterol.

Calcium loss: Meat protein is acid-forming in the body, creating an ideal environment for bacteria to breed and diseases to take a hold. Calcium (an alkalizing agent) is required to neutralize the pH in the blood, which can cause calcium imbalance and increase the risk of bone loss (see pages 225 on Osteoporosis).

What Kind of Proteins Should You Eat?

The best protein sources do not necessarily have the highest quantity: the quality of the protein is crucial.

Look for good quality and bioavailabilty. Animal products though high in protein, are also high in saturated fats and the protein is harder to assimilate. And the quality of the meat could be full of antibiotics, growth hormones and pesticides.

Complete vs. Incomplete Protein. A complete protein source contains all eight essential amino acids. Though animal proteins are a complete protein source, they cause the blood to be acidic and thicken.

Plant protein is incomplete but preferred over animal protein. Being incomplete means that you need to eat a wider variety in order to obtain all eight essential amino acids. Some of the most complete plant protein sources are quinoa, avocado, spirulina and chlorella (see Plant Based Protein Chart on page 134).

2. CARBOHYDRATES: *Starches & Sugars* (125)

Starches and sugars come under the classification, carbohydrates, in the FDA standard for food groups. These provide the principle source of food energy. Carbohydrates are needed as fuel for muscular work and physical activity. Excess sugars and starches that are not utilized as energy are transformed by the body chemistry into fat and stored in the least active body parts, causing obesity.

Carbohydrates originate in plants as sugars created by photosynthesis, then are formed into clusters as starches. Consumed by humans, they are broken down by your body's metabolism into simple sugar – glucose – for use by body cells. It's important to eat only natural sugar starches and avoid all refined GMO white/wheat flours, sugars, etc.

Natural starches and sugars are found in all fresh fruits and vegetables, honey, pure maple syrup, sorghum, Stevia and blackstrap molasses, organic whole grains and their flours (barley, oats, quinoa, millet, amaranth, rye, etc.), beans, lentils and peas, organic brown rice and potatoes. In fact, all natural foods contain some carbohydrates.

Modern GMO Wheat – No Longer Mother Nature's Wheat!!!

Modern GMO wheat isn't really the wheat that Mother Nature intended. About 700 million tons of wheat are grown worldwide making it second most-produced grain after corn. It's grown on more land area than any other commercial crop and considered a staple food for humans.

The Wheat We Eat Today Isn't the Wheat Our Grandmothers Ate!

The balance and ratio of nutrients "Mother Nature" created for wheat has been modified! At some point in our history, this ancient grain was nutritious, however modern GMO wheat really isn't the same wheat at all. Once agribusiness took over to develop a higher-yielding crop, wheat became hybridized to the extent it has completely transformed from its prehistorical genetic configuration.

The majority of wheat is processed into 60% extraction or bleached white flour. The standard for most wheat products means that 40% of the original wheat grain is removed! So not only do we have an unhealthier, modified, and hybridized strain of wheat, we also remove and further degrade its nutritional value by processing it!

Unfortunately, the 40% that gets removed includes the bran and the germ of the wheat grain – its most nutrient-rich parts. In the process of making 60% extraction flour, over half of the vitamins B1, B2, B3, E, folic acid, calcium, phosphorus, zinc, copper, iron, and fiber are lost. Any processed foods with GMO wheat are unhealthy since they cause more body health risks than benefits.

Heavily marketed white carbs (white sugar, flour, pasta, etc.) that are packaged in boxes are designed to make you crave more. They're not good for your body, your mind or your soul! – BetterNutrition.com

---

Seek out and choose from whole foods: organic fruits, vegetables, rice, beans, nuts, seeds, etc. rather than the commercial, refined white flour and sugar products and other highly processed canned goods in center aisles.

People who turn away from GMO wheat have dropped substantial weight. Even diabetics no longer become diabetic; people with arthritis have dramatic relief; and less acid reflux; leg swelling; and irritable bowel syndrome.

"The whiter the bread, the sooner you're dead!" The body doesn't recognize processed GMO wheat as food. Nutrient absorption from processed wheat products is thus consequential with almost no nutritional value.

Even if you choose 100% whole wheat products they are based on modern GMO wheat strains created by irradiation of wheat seeds and embryos with chemicals, gamma rays, and high-dose X-rays to induce mutations. You're still consuming genetically modified grain.

To avoid these toxic wheat-oriented products, we suggest eating "real food," organic whole grain products made with non-GMO organic grains.

Health Problems Associated With GMO Wheat

Dr. Marcia Alvarez who specializes in nutritional programs for obese patients says, "**Modern GMO wheat grains could certainly be considered as the root of all evil in the world of nutrition** since they cause so many documented health problems across so many populations in the world." See web: *NonGMOproject.org*

Dr. Alvarez asserted that GMO wheat is now responsible for more intolerances than almost any other food in the world! *"In my practice of over two decades, we have documented that for every ten people with digestive problems, obesity, irritable bowel syndrome, diabetes, arthritis and even heart disease, 8 out of 10 people have health problems with wheat. Once we remove GMO wheat from their diets, most of their symptoms disappear within three to six months,"* she added. Dr. Alvarez estimates that between the coming influx of genetically modified (GMO) strains of wheat and current growing tendency of wheat elimination worldwide, a trend is emerging in the next 20 years that will likely see 80% of people stop their consumption of GMO wheat in any form!

If you select 100% organic whole wheat products, the bran and germ of the wheat will remain in the product, and the health benefits will be impressive! Organic non-GMO whole wheat is a good dietary fiber source.

Fiber is vital for good health, healthy elimination and adequate intake helps prevent colon cancer! Everyone will benefit from making sure they regularly include foods in their diet such as organic non-GMO whole grains, barley, oats, beans, fruits and vegetables that provide healthy fibers.

3. FATS: *Can Be Healthy or Unhealthy*

Fat is also an important source of dietary energy. It has more than twice the energy value of the same amount of carbohydrates or protein. As already pointed out a certain amount of fat is part of a healthy diet. Let us remind you that your fat intake should ideally consist of only unsaturated fats. The saturated fats in meat, eggs, poultry and dairy products (see pages 31-33) often are best avoided or kept to a minimum. It is these saturated fats which can overload your body with excess cholesterol.

The Function of Fat in the Body

Our nerves, muscles and organs must be *cushioned* by a normal amount of fat. If we did not have a certain amount of fat in our *gluteus maximus* (the buttocks), for example, we would never be able to sit down because we would have to sit directly on our bones and muscles.

Those who wish to lose weight should reduce the *saturated fat* content of their diet, and those who wish to gain should increase their *good, unsaturated fat* intake. But even when on a reducing diet, there should be some fat in your diet because it plays an essential role in your body's chemistry! Stored in the body, fat provides a source of heat and energy, while the accumulation of a certain amount of fat around the vital organs (such as the kidneys) gives great protection against cold and injury.

Fat also has a function to perform in the body's cells, for which special fats known as unsaturated fatty acids are needed in small amounts. Without these a roughness or scaliness of the skin would result. Fats have another all-important main function: they carry the fat-soluble vitamins A, D, E and K through the body. As you can see, a certain amount of fat in the diet is necessary to a healthy functioning body. But it's the kind of fat that is most important! *Unsaturated fat is best. Caution: – it is wise to go light on the clogging saturated fats!*

Dr. Dean Ornish has been able to reverse heart disease in more than 70% of patients who follow, among other things, a low-fat, vegetarian diet.

There are dozens of foods that contain almost NO bad fat. Healthy avocados and olives, organic fruits and vegetables have good fat!

128

Unsaturated Fats Are Best for Heart Health

There are actually two types of unsaturated fats – *polyunsaturated* and *monounsaturated*, both of which are liquid at room temperature. Two types of polyunsaturated fats – omega-3 and omega-6 fatty acids – cannot be produced by the human body, but play an essential role in brain development, skin and hair growth, maintaining a healthy reproductive system and in regulating our metabolism. Plus, both types promote coronary health by lowering "bad" LDL cholesterol and raising "good" HDL cholesterol. To increase your intake of unsaturated fats, try replacing other fatty foods with these 4 items:

1. Olive Oil: is full of healthy unsaturated fats. 1 Tbsp. of olive oil has almost 12 grams of unsaturated fat and only 2 grams of saturated. In addition, olive oil provides a heart-friendly dose of both omega-3 and omega-6 fatty acids. Mix organic olive oil with organic apple cider vinegar to create a delicious healthy salad dressing or use it to sauté your veggies. Olive oil is great for cooking, but should not be used for deep frying.

2. Almonds: Healthy raw nuts and their butter with beneficial unsaturated fats. Not only are they a good source of monounsaturated and polyunsaturated fatty acids, they also provide Vitamin E, which is great for hair, nails and skin.

3. Peanut Butter: Pick organic all-natural, non-GMO peanut butter, and make sure there is nothing in the ingredient list that includes the word hydrogenated. Avoid any jars with trans-fat on the nutrition label, as these are most harmful to the body. To make your own nut butters see page 130.

4. Avocados: are full of good unsaturated fats, low in saturated fat, which help lower the risk of heart disease. Their smooth creamy texture makes them a great replacement for mayonnaise or cheese. For parties, mash avocados together with small amounts: onion, garlic, and diced tomato . . . makes a tasty guacamole!

A Massachusetts Medical Society Study showed that using extra virgin olive oil lowers the need for blood pressure medication. The ones who used olive oil reduced their blood pressure medication by 50%! Olive oil enhances heart health by lowering "bad" cholesterol without affecting "good" HDL.

Organic Extra-Virgin Olive Oil is Highly Recommended

Mother Nature has provided us with wonderful healthy oils which can be used in preparing foods, salad dressings or for sautéing and marinating. Virgin, cold-pressed olive oil has been used for centuries. Even Hippocrates used olive oil in his practice. Try organic extra virgin (first pressed) olive oil – it's the healthiest of oils!

Other healthy oils are cold-pressed safflower, sesame, sunflower and soybean oils. These oils can be used in salad dressings, recipes, baking, etc. We still use oils sparingly. They're healthy in polyunsaturated and unsaturated fatty acids. Please, don't use genetically engineered canola oil.

Another favorite of ours is organic unrefined flaxseed oil which is the richest source of omega-3 essential fatty acids (more than double that of fish oils). We prefer whole flaxseeds, you can grind them in a coffee grinder as needed and sprinkle over breakfast cereals, oatmeal and smoothies. We also use hemp seed oil. These two fragile oils must be kept cold and refrigerated once opened for safety and never heated as they are easily oxidized and damaged by heat and light. You can add them to foods after they have been cooked. We suggest you add 1-2 tsps. of these oils to your diet daily, or grind seeds for healthy omega fatty acids which are vital to bodily functions, especially the heart (for more info on EFA and Omega-3 see page 227).

130

How To Make Healthy Nut Butters

Grind 1 $^1/_2$ cups of raw unsalted organic nuts of your choice in a food processor or blender. Keep grinding nuts down until they are a thick, fudge-like paste. Then add sunflower or nut oil (start with 1 Tbsp. and add more only if necessary for desired thickness). Blend until smooth. Best kept refrigerated.

Organic natural foods are the greatest source for staying healthy!
– Patricia Bragg, Pioneer Health Crusader

The Bragg Healthy Lifestyle helps make a healthier you & a healthier world!

Raw Nuts and Seeds are Healthy Foods

Gary Null, a leading health activist writes in his book, *Complete Guide to Sensible Eating*, raw nuts and seeds are good sources of protein, minerals (especially magnesium), some B vitamins and unsaturated fatty acids (pages 134, 214-215). They are delicious snack foods or used with other foods. There are few foods that are more highly packed with life force than raw seeds and nuts.

Flax and Chia are Seeds for Life

Flaxseeds are packed with omega-3, lignans, protein and fiber, which are natural antioxidants. Omega-3 helps remove toxins and helps prevent heart disease (page 227) and the lignans aid in preventing cancers. Each Tbsp of flax contains about 8 grams of fiber that helps fight "bad" cholesterol and type 2 diabetes. Flaxseed improves conditions from cardiac and autoimmune functions to allergies and digestion. Other benefits include: healthier skin, hair and nails; 40-60% improvement in athletic performance; enhanced learning ability; and better brain function. Whole flax and chia seeds can be stored for months in an airtight container in a cool, dark place. **Then enjoy as needed. You can grind them in coffee grinder.**

131

Chia Seeds are also rich in omega-3 fatty acids and antioxidants! Chia seeds provide fiber, as well as calcium, phosphorus, magnesium, iron, niacin and zinc. They can slow down how fast our bodies convert carbohydrates into simple sugars, which may have great benefits for diabetics.

Chia seeds have a nutlike flavor. They are tasty, delicious and nutritious. You can sprinkle whole or ground chia and flax seeds on cereals, yogurt, salads, soups and veggies. Also add to prepared smoothies, infant formulas, baby foods and nutrition bars! You can even add them into flour when making baked goods such as cookies, muffins, etc.

Make this ACV-Flaxseed Bowel Lubricant Cleanse Tea

Boil 2 cups distilled water with 4 Tbsps whole flaxseeds for 15 minutes or soak overnight. (Mixture becomes jelly-like when cold.) Stir 2 Tbsps of this mixture, plus 1 tsp ACV in 8 oz. distilled (hot or cold) water. Add maple syrup or honey if desired. Drink upon arising and an hour before bed. Store mixture in refrigerator and use when needed.

Dr. Charles Attwood – Great Health Crusader

As a Doctor, Humanitarian, Dedicated Health Crusader, Devoted Pediatrician for over 40 years, and Fellow of the American Academy of Pediatrics, Dr. Charles Raymond Attwood fought many battles against mainstream medicine and big business to ensure the health of people everywhere, particularly children. He championed a low-fat vegetarian menu for children, was a strong health and nutrition activist and an associate of Dr. Benjamin Spock. One major battle occurred in 1996. As a member of the Center for Science in the Public Interest, Dr. Attwood led opposition to the giant Gerber Baby Food Company's practice of diluting its baby foods with water, sugar and starch. He won! Gerber stopped this 40 year crime against America's children. Now their foods are 100% fruits and vegetables. Other baby food companies then followed. See web: *VegSource.com.*

Dr. Charles Attwood held high the banner advocating a low-fat, plant-based diet as the most healthy for youngsters. His highly praised 1995 book, *Low-fat Prescription for Kids* makes a strong scientific argument for this diet! His research shows how to avoid the leading causes of premature death later as adults (heart disease, stroke, cancers and diabetes). It's important for children and adults alike to follow his program.

132

Dr. Attwood's Tips for Low-Fat Shopping

- Spend most of your time in the produce department.
- Try new varieties of produce. Look at those with the most intense colors and remember organic is best!
- Don't forget about pasta made from rice or quinoa.
- Buy unrefined, sugarless, high-fiber rice or oat cereals.
- When buying packaged, canned, frozen foods, read labels.
- Don't underestimate beans – whether dried, frozen or canned, they are delicious and healthy for you.
- Buy low- or no-fat healthy snacks – there are many choices. Careful, as some are high in salt, sugar and calories.
- Replace milk and low-fat dairy products with nut, oat or rice milks and tofu cheeses.

Eliminating Meat is Safer and Healthier

Play it safe, become a healthy vegetarian! Look what they put in cattle feed and in some cases dog and cat foods – the dead, ground-up carcasses of other feed lot animals who didn't make it to the slaughterhouse.

Speaking of the slaughterhouse scene, what kind of chemical reaction do you suppose would occur in your body if somebody put a choke chain around your neck to keep you in line, shoved you onto a conveyor belt, and made you watch in horror as all of those in line in front of you were beheaded one by one? Well, your body would be pumped so full of adrenaline from all that fear you wouldn't know what hit you! All that unused adrenaline is extremely toxic! If you think for a minute that most of the meat that you consume is not packed with this toxic substance, you are sadly mistaken!

Also, consider the fact that cattle, sheep, chickens, et al, are all vegetarians. When you eat them, you are just eating polluted vegetables! Why not skip all the waste and toxins and just eat healthy, organic vegetables?

And what about that myth that you have to eat meat to get your protein? If that were true, where do you suppose farm animals, especially horses, get their protein? They are vegetarians! They get their protein from the grains and grasses that they eat. You are no different. You can get proteins you need from a wide variety of organic whole grains, tofu, raw nuts, seeds, beans, fruits and vegetables that Mother Nature put on this planet for your health. Study the *Plant Based Protein Chart on next page.*

Beware of Too Much Protein in Middle-Age: *Study in "Cell Metabolism Journal" has showed that high protein consumption (such as red meat) is linked to an increased risk of cancer, diabetes and death in middle-aged adults. In fact, a high-protein diet is nearly as bad as smoking for your health. A survey revealed that those aged 50+ who ate a high-protein diet (20% of calories consumed came from protein), were four times more likely to die from cancer, diabetes and kidney disease in the following 18 years. These effects either reduced or disappeared among participants when their high-protein diet switched to plant-based.*

Research has shown that by simply eating nuts you can improve your blood-lipid profiles (cholesterol & triglyceride levels), to significantly reduce your risk of heart disease and lose weight. – Dr. David Williams, "Guide to Healthy Living"

Copy page and share with family, friends, etc.

Plant-Based Protein Chart

BEANS & LEGUMES

(1 cup cooked)	PROTEIN IN GRAMS
Soybeans	29
Lentils	18
Adzuki Beans	17
Cannellini	17
Navy Beans	16
Split Peas	16
Black Beans	15
Garbanzos (chick peas)	15
Kidney Beans	15
Great Northern Beans	15
Lima Beans	15
Black-eyed Peas	14
Pinto Beans	14
Mung Beans	14
Tofu (3 oz.)	7 to 12
Green Peas (whole)	9

RAW NUTS & SEEDS

(1/4 cup or 4 Tbsps)	PROTEIN IN GRAMS
Chia Seeds	12
Macadamia Nuts	11
Flax Seeds	8
Sunflower Seeds	8
Almonds	7
Pumpkin Seeds	7
Sesame Seeds	7
Walnuts	5
Brazil Nuts	5
Hazelnuts	5
Pine Nuts	4
Cashews	4

134

NUT BUTTERS

(2 Tbsps)	PROTEIN IN GRAMS
Peanut Butter	7 to 9
Almond Butter	5 to 8
Cashew Butter	4 to 5
Sesame - Tahini	6

VEGETABLES

(1 Serving or 1 cup)	PROTEIN IN GRAMS
Spirulina	8.6
Corn (1 cob)	5
Potato (with skin)	5
Mushrooms, Oyster	5
Artichoke (1 medium)	4
Collard Greens	4
Broccoli	4
Brussel Sprouts	4
Mushrooms, Shiitake	3.5
Swiss Chard	3
Kale	2.5
Asparagus (5 spears)	2
String Beans	2
Beets	2
Peas	2
Sweet Potato	3
Summer Squash	2
Cabbage	2
Carrot	2
Cauliflower	2
Squash	2
Celery	1
Spinach	1
Bell Peppers	1
Cucumber	1
Eggplant	1
Leeks	1
Lettuce	1
Tomato (1 medium)	1
Radish	1
Turnips	1

DAIRY & NUT MILKS

(1 cup)	PROTEIN IN GRAMS
Oat Milk	3 to 4
Almond Milk	1 to 2
Rice Milk	1
Eggs (1) *(free-range)*	6

FRUITS

(1 Serving or 1 cup)	PROTEIN IN GRAMS
Avocado (1 medium)	4
Banana (1)	1 to 2
Blackberries (1 cup)	2
Pomegranate (1)	1.5
Blueberries (1 cup)	1
Cantaloupe (1 cup)	1
Cherries (1 cup)	1
Grapes (1 cup)	1
Honeydew (1 cup)	1
Kiwi (1 large)	1
Lemon (1)	1
Mango (1)	1
Nectarine (1)	1
Orange (1)	1
Peach (1)	1
Pear (1)	1
Pineapple (1 cup)	1
Plum (1)	1
Raspberries (1 cup)	1
Strawberries (1 cup)	1
Watermelon (1 cup)	1

GRAINS & RICE

(1 cup cooked)	PROTEIN IN GRAMS
Triticale	25
Millet	8.4
Amaranth	7
Oat Bran	7
Wild Rice	7
Couscous (whole wheat)	6
Bulgur Wheat	6
Buckwheat	6
Teff	6
Oat Groats	6
Barley	5
Quinoa	5
Brown Rice	5
Spelt	5

This chart displays protein content of common vegetarian foods.
Note that in order to determine amount of protein that is optimal for your body, use the following formula that is based on a vegan diet: *RDA recommends that we take in 0.36 grams of protein per pound that we weigh* (100 lbs. x 0.36 = 36 grams).
Data from webs: *TheHolyKale.com* • *VegParadise.com* • *vrg.org (Vegetarian Resource Group).*

Meat: Bad Fat, Toxic Uric Acid & Cholesterol

Meat is a major source of toxic uric acid and cholesterol, both harmful to your health! **If you eat meat, it should be an organically fed source.** Fresh fish can be less toxic than flesh proteins, but beware, as fish from polluted waters can be loaded with mercury, lead, cadmium, DDT, radiation and other toxins. If unsure of the safety of waters the fish come from, don't risk it!

Avoid shellfish – shrimp, lobster, crayfish! If you choose to eat fish, shop for wild-caught, low mercury varieties such as salmon, sea bass and halibut.

Don't eat pork or pork products! Pigs are the only animals besides man that develop arteriosclerosis.

We feel that *meat and dairy products* are far more dangerous than they are healthy! Meats are high in visible fat, cholesterol and toxins from the animal. That's why we stress to meat eaters not to have meat more than 1-2 times a week and always trim off fat before cooking. Placing meat on a rack during cooking, baking or broiling helps drain off most of the fat and keeps it from soaking in its own unhealthy grease and drippings.

135

Don't eat greasy fried foods. The frying pan is the cradle of indigestion, heart disease and death!

Poultry – chicken and turkey – the organically fed and hormone and drug free are safer animal proteins. Most poultry is commercially mass fed and heavily drugged with antibiotics and hormones! Discard all poultry skins and giblets because they are high in fat.

Eggs. If you do eat eggs, limit to no more than four per week. Remember, yolks contain high cholesterol fat. Fertile fresh eggs from free-range, organic fed chickens are best.

However, every body is different, and as you follow *The Bragg Healthy Lifestyle* and experience radiant health, you will discover what foods your body needs. If you choose to eat animal protein, make sure you're buying hormone- and antibiotic-free chicken, beef or turkey, and wild-caught fish. Avoid high-mercury species/types such as tuna, opting instead for salmon, sardines, and scallops. Quality is the most significant factor in eating animal protein.

4. FRUITS & VEGETABLES: *Miracle Foods*

Three-fifths of your diet should consist of organic, raw and lightly cooked vegetables and fresh fruits. These natural miracle foods not only contribute phytonutrients (see chart page 140), isoflavones, vitamins and organic minerals to the diet, but they also add bulk and moisture required for healthy elimination and smooth body functioning. They also help maintain the alkaline reserve of the body and add variety, color, flavor and texture to the diet.

Vegetables are virtually fat-free and contain no cholesterol!

The ideal way to get the full amount of vitamins and minerals from organic vegetables is in their raw state, in fresh vegetable salads or as garnishes with meals. When cooking vegetables some vitamins and minerals may be lost.

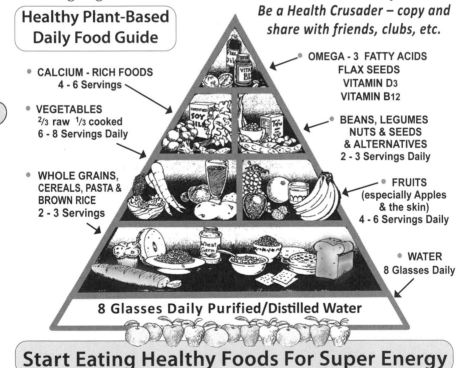

Healthy Plant-Based Daily Food Guide

Be a Health Crusader – copy and share with friends, clubs, etc.

- OMEGA - 3 FATTY ACIDS
  FLAX SEEDS
  VITAMIN D3
  VITAMIN B12

- CALCIUM - RICH FOODS
  4 - 6 Servings

- VEGETABLES
  ⅔ raw ⅓ cooked
  6 - 8 Servings Daily

- BEANS, LEGUMES
  NUTS & SEEDS
  & ALTERNATIVES
  2 - 3 Servings Daily

- WHOLE GRAINS,
  CEREALS, PASTA &
  BROWN RICE
  2 - 3 Servings

- FRUITS
  (especially Apples
  & the skin)
  4 - 6 Servings Daily

- WATER
  8 Glasses Daily

8 Glasses Daily Purified/Distilled Water

136

Start Eating Healthy Foods For Super Energy

This ***Healthy Plant-Based Daily Food Guide Pyramid*** illustration represents an ideal way of eating for achieving optimal nutrition, health and wellness. You will notice that this Food Guide Pyramid is based on healthy organic plant foods, with emphasis on purified water, fruits, vegetables, whole grains, vegetable protein foods, non-dairy calcium foods, raw nuts and seeds. Eating a diet based on these dietary guidelines will help you get the nutrients needed for optimal health. It's not only the best diet for wellness, disease prevention and longevity, it also provides the right balance for building a healthy heart.

Purified/Distilled Water: The pyramid's foundation is purified water. We recommend drinking *pure distilled water* as it is best water for the body! ***Drink at least eight – 8 oz glasses of distilled water daily and even more if your lifestyle (sports and/or work) requires it.***

Whole Grains: Whole grains are the next pyramid level. Avoid all processed, GMO refined grain products and eat only unrefined, organic whole grain bread and cereal products! Grains such as quinoa, whole wheat, brown rice, barley, oats, millet, kamut as well as 100% whole grain breads and cereals are best! One serving of whole grains is equal to 1 slice whole grain bread, 1 ounce ready-to-eat whole grain cereal, 1 cup cooked whole grains such as brown rice, oatmeal or other grains, 1 cup 100% whole wheat (or other whole grains) pasta or noodles, and 1 ounce of other whole grain products. ***We recommend 1-3 servings of organic, non-GMO whole grains daily.***

Vegetables: We recommend eating as many of your vegetables organic and raw (uncooked, in salads, juices, smoothies, etc.) as possible! When cooking vegetables, don't overcook them! Steaming or lightly stir-frying is best.

137

The more colorful rainbow of vegetables is better for your health as they contain more valuable nutrients and healthful phytonutrients (see page 139-141). Eat a wide variety of organic vegetables daily. One vegetable serving is equal to 1 cup cooked vegetables or 1 cup raw uncooked vegetables, 1 cup salad, or 3/4 cup vegetable juice. ***We recommend having 6-8 or more vegetable servings daily.***

Fruits: Like vegetables, the more colorful the fruits the better they are for you! Have organic fruits as much as possible! One serving of fruit is equal to 1 medium apple, banana, orange, pear or other fruit, 1/2 cup fruit, 1/2 cup of fruit juice or 1/4 cup dried fruit. ***We recommend eating 4-6 servings or more of organic fruits daily.***

Grains that are heart-healthy are organic brown rice, organic whole grain breads, cereals, and pastas. Also popcorn, organic corn is a whole grain. Our favorite is air-popped and top with coconut aminos, olive oil and good quality nutritional yeast (recipe page 150). There's also buckwheat, barley, millet, and tasty quinoa is a complete protein and makes an ideal breakfast cereal.

Calcium-Rich Foods: Are plant-derived calcium-rich foods. Plant sources of calcium are healthier than dairy products because they don't contain saturated fats or cholesterol. Health calcium-rich foods are: oat milk, tofu, broccoli and green leafy vegetables. Examples of serving sizes of plant-derived calcium-rich foods include: $1/2$ cup tofu, $1/3$ cup almonds, 1 cup cooked or 2 cups high calcium dark greens (kale, collards, broccoli, bok choy or other Chinese greens), 1 cup calcium-rich beans (white, navy, Great Northern), $1/2$ cup seaweed, 1 Tbsb blackstrap molasses, 5 or more figs. *We recommend having 4-6 servings of healthy non-dairy sources of calcium rich foods daily.*

Beans, Legumes, Nuts & Seeds: These are the healthy protein foods. Vegetable protein foods are more optimal compared to animal protein foods. Vegetable proteins do not contain the artery clogging saturated fats and cholesterol found in animal foods. They also contain protective factors to prevent heart disease, cancer and diabetes. Vegetable proteins are high quality and provide the body with the essential amino acids that it requires. One serving of vegetable protein foods include: 1 cup cooked legumes (beans, lentils, dried peas), $1/2$ cup firm tofu or tempeh, 1 serving of "veggie meat" alternate (e.g. veggie burger patty or meatless meat), 3 tablespoons nut or seed butter, 1 cup soy milk. *We recommend you have 2 to 3 or more vegetable protein servings daily with meals.*

Healthy Fats, Essential Fatty Acids, Omega-3 and Other Nutrients: Servings of healthy fats include: 1 tsp of flaxseed oil, 1 Tbsp of Organic Olive Oil, 3 tsps of raw walnuts or pumpkin seeds. Other healthy essential nutrients include: ground flaxseeds or chia seeds and nutritional B-Complex supplements that provide vitamin B12. Do provide your body with nutritional supplements your body requires for optimal health.

138

The chemistry of food a person eats becomes his own body chemistry. Perhaps the most valuable result of all education is the ability to inspire and make yourself do the thing you have to do, when it ought to be done, as it ought to be done, whether you like to do it or not! – Patricia Bragg, Pioneer Health Crusader

---

Coconut oil is about 90% saturated fat, but contains a fat called lauric acid, which your body processes faster and more efficiently than the saturated fat in a T-bone steak (look for organic virgin coconut oil). Avoid anything that says "partially hydrogenated." – DoctorOz.com

What are Nature's Miracle Phytonutrients?

These wonderful, organic compounds are found in plants, ('phyto' means 'plant' in Greek), and are vital to human health. Increasingly, scientific studies are showing that phytonutrients help protect us from many serious health issues, including heart disease and stroke. Organic fruits, vegetables, grains, legumes, nuts and some teas are rich in these miracle phytonutrients.

Physicians and Scientists have written about the critical nature of these foods for thousands of years, but the specific benefits of phytonutrients are still being discovered. They are created when plants absorb energy from the earth, water, air and sun. This energy helps plants survive environmental challenges such as diseases, damage, drought, excessive heat, ultraviolet sunrays and poisons. This incredible energy forms an important part of the plant's immune system! It appears to provide humans with the same benefits, when we consume the plants. They help increase our immune and regeneration systems. They give us strength, endurance, and ultimately help us feel better and live longer.

Health Benefits of Phytonutrients

The body must have these phytonutrients and enzymes to break down food, kill viruses and bacteria and dissolve tumors! A diet of at least 50% raw, unprocessed foods is vital to make sure that we are getting enough enzymes and phytonutrients to optimize the body's processes.

Plants contain more than 10,000 phytonutrients, one reason 10-14 servings of fruits and veggies daily are recommended. Plants and vegetables contain different phytonutrients, having a variety in your diet is important.

On an average, the plant foods have 64 times more antioxidants than animal foods, which is critical to understand because when it comes to antioxidants, the more we eat, the more our health benefits. Eating a diet high in antioxidants (see page 29) is important for several reasons, including the fact it appears to reduce inflammation in the body (see pages 52-54). See chart on next page for health benefits of different plant sources.

Mother Nature's Miracle Phytonutrients Help Prevent Cancer:

Make sure to get your daily dose of naturally occurring, cancer-fighting super foods – Phytonutrients are abundant in apples, tomatoes, onions, garlic, beans, legumes, soybeans, cabbage, cauliflower, broccoli, citrus, etc. Champions with highest count of Phytonutrients – apples and tomatoes.

Phytonutrient	Food Sources	Health Action
PHYTOESTROGEN ISOFLAVONES	*Soy products, flaxseed, seeds and nuts, yams, alfalfa, pomegranates lentils, carrots, apples*	*Helps block some cancers, aids in menopausal symptoms, balances hormones, helps improve memory, enhances heart health*
PHYTOSTEROLS	*Plant oils: corn, sesame, safflower; rice bran, wheat germ, peanuts*	*Blocks hormonal role in cancers, inhibits uptake of cholesterol from diet, reduce risk of heart attack*
LIGNANS	*Flaxseeds, rye, lentils, soy mushrooms, barley*	*Helps prevent breast cancer, heart disease and balances hormones*
SAPONINS	*Yams, beets, beans, cabbage, nuts, soybeans*	*Helps prevent cancer cells from multiplying, reduces cholesterol*
TERPENES	*Carrots, winter squash, sweet potatoes, yams, apples, cantaloupes, cherries*	*Antioxidants – protects DNA from free radical-induced damage, and improves immunity*
	Tomatoes and its sauces, tomato-based products	*Helps block UVA & UVB and offers help to protect against cancers – breast, prostate, etc.*
	Spinach, kale, beet and turnip greens, cabbage	*Protects eyes from macular degeneration,*
	Red chile peppers	*Keeps carcinogens from binding to DNA*
QUERCETIN (& FLAVONOIDS)	*Apples (especially the skins), red onions and green tea*	*Strong cancer fighter, protects heart - arteries. Reduces pain, allergy and asthma symptoms*
	Citrus fruits (flavonoids)	*Promotes protective enzymes*
PHENOLS	*Apples, fennel, parsley, carrots, alfalfa, cabbage*	*Helps prevent blood clotting & has important anticancer properties*
	Cinnamon	*Promotes healthy blood sugar and glucose metabolism*
	Citrus fruits, broccoli, cabbage, cucumbers, green peppers, tomatoes	*Antioxidants – flavonoids, block membrane receptor sites for certain hormones*
	Apples, grape seeds	*Strong antioxidants; fights germs and bacteria, strengthens immune system, veins and capillaries*
	Grapes, especially skins	*Antioxidant, antimutagen; promotes detoxification. Acts as carcinogen inhibitors*
	Yellow and green squash	*Antihepatotoxic, antitumor*
SULFUR COMPOUNDS	*Onions and garlic, (fresh is always best) Red onions (our favorite) also contain Quercetin Onions help keep doctor away*	*Promotes liver enzymes, inhibits cholesterol synthesis, reduces triglycerides, lowers blood pressure improves immune response, fights infections, germs and parasites*

Main Sources of Phytonutrients

The following are high in phytonutrients: carrots and yellow vegetables (sweet potatoes and pumpkins), peaches, apricots, broccoli, leafy greens (kale, spinach, turnip greens), tomatoes, pink grapefruit, watermelon, guava, blackberries, walnuts, strawberries, cranberries, raspberries, blueberries, grape juice, and prunes, red cabbage, pineapple, oranges, plums, pinto beans, spinach, kiwi fruit and red peppers.

The more live, unprocessed foods we eat the more phytonutrients and enzymes we consume the healthier our diet. This natural food is full of energy we need to live longer, healthier lives! To boost your immune system and cell regeneration of the body, eat more phytonutrients, practice deep breathing exercises daily, get physical exercise, and make sure that your diet is at least 50% raw, unprocessed, natural organic foods. That's The Bragg Healthy Lifestyle.

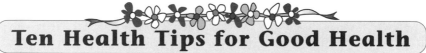

Ten Health Tips for Good Health

- *Respect and protect your body as the highest manifestation of your life.*
- *Abstain from unnatural, devitalized foods and stimulating beverages.*
- *Nourish your body with only natural unprocessed, live foods.*
- *Extend your years in health for loving, sharing and charitable service.*
- *Regenerate your body by the right balance of activity and rest.*
- *Purify your cells, tissue and blood with healthy organic foods, and with pure water, clean air and gentle sunshine.*
- *Abstain from all food when out of sorts in mind or body.*
- *Keep thoughts, words and emotions pure, calm, loving and uplifting.*
- *Increase your knowledge of Mother Nature's Laws, follow them, and enjoy the fruits of your life's labor.*
- *Lift up yourself, friends and family by loyal obedience to Mother Nature's and God's Healthy, Natural Laws of Living.*

Bragg Healthy Lifestyle Plan

- *Read, plan, plot, and follow through for supreme health and longevity.*
- *Underline, highlight or dog-ear pages as you read important passages.*
- *Organizing your lifestyle helps you identify what's important in your life.*
- *Be faithful to your health goals everyday for a healthy, long, happy life.*
- *Where space allows we have included "words of wisdom" from great minds to motivate and inspire you. Please share your favorite sayings with us.*
- *Write us about your successes following The Bragg Healthy Lifestyle.*

Warning! – Avoid All Unhealthy Microwaved Foods

In the past 40 years (health destroying) microwaves have practically replaced traditional methods of cooking, especially with *on-the-go people* of today's world. But how much do you really know about them? A Swiss Study found that food which is microwaved is not the food it was before! The microwave radiation deforms and destroys the molecular structure of the food – creating radiolytic compounds! When microwaved food is eaten, abnormal changes then occur in your blood and immune systems! These include a decrease in hemoglobin and white blood cell counts and increase in cholesterol levels! An article in *Pediatrics Journal* warns microwaving human milk damages the anti-infective properties it usually gives to a mother's baby! Research done at the University of Warwick in Great Britain warns that microwave radiation is damaging to the vital electromagnetic activity of human life vibrations! Over 20 years ago Russia established wise microwave radiation limits more stringent than the United States and Great Britain! Beware – don't use microwaves!!

142

Avoid Refined, Processed, Unhealthy Foods!

Eliminate refined, white flour products and white sugar products entirely. Eat no mushy, dead, refined cereals or those dry sugared cereals, that are unhealthy despite some being enriched with chemically produced vitamins and minerals. (Health Stores carry natural organic whole-grains, cereals, granola, breads, rolls, pastas, even pastries.)

Avoid these foods: Fried, salted, refined, preserved and chemicalized foods; coffee, black (caffeinated) teas, cola, soft drinks, sugared drinks and alcohol drinks; overcooked, over-salted vegetables and salted, creamed and white flour-thickened soups. Please read page 144 for a complete foods-to-avoid list for alert wise healthy buying.

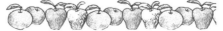

You can be a sewage system when eating unhealthy, highly processed foods.
Remember, live foods produce healthy, live people!

USA leads the world in heart disease, strokes, cancer and diabetes! Why?
It's our fast junk foods, high sugars, fats, milk and processed foods diet!

You now know the foods to avoid: Refined, unhealthy foods high in fat, salt and sugar; meat and dairy products; sugared foods and beverages and chemicalized water.

You now know the foods you can eat: Fresh fruits (organically grown is always best to buy or grow yourself); fresh juices; raw salads; fresh vegetables – raw, steamed, baked or stir-fryed; vegetable proteins, beans, legumes, tofu, raw nuts, seeds, etc. If you really want animal and fish proteins, limit to twice weekly. Occasionally, eat nothing but fresh fruits, raw vegetables and sprouts for 1 or 2 days a week. Remember, vegetarians are healthiest among Americans! World research proves this! See web: *www.Ornish.com*

Use your imagination to plan enjoyable, live food meals that are powerful for super health! Keep meals simple! Avoid eating too many food mixtures. Don't overeat! Be moderate in all things for best health! Eat only when you are really hungry, not because it is mealtime. Earn your food by activity, vigorous exercise and deep breathing. You will see how much more you really enjoy food when you deserve and earn it!

Stevia – The Natural Herbal Sweetener

Stevia is an herb native to South America (*stevia.com*). It's widely grown for its sweet leaves. In its unprocessed form it is 30-times sweeter than sugar. It is a low carbohydrate, low-sugar food alternative. Stevia shows promise for treating such conditions as obesity and high blood pressure. It does not effect blood sugar and it even enhances glucose tolerance. Stevia is a safe, delicious, health sweetener for diabetics. Children can use Stevia without concerns, as it does not cause cavities.

If just half of the billions of dollars spent on cancer research were spent on educating the public on how to avoid disease – millions of lives would be saved from cancer. – Joel Fuhrman, M.D., "Fasting & Eating for Health"

Junk foods, processed meats, hot dogs, sausage, sugar and fast foods can increase inflammation in your body which could lead to chronic disease. – Dr. Bob Martin, author of "Secret Nerve Cures"
• www.DoctorBob.com

Millions of Americans are committing slow suicide with their unhealthy lifestyle: meat eating, high sugar and fat diets, smoking, drinking, drugs – all damage their organs and arteries. – Patricia Bragg, Pioneer Health Crusader

Avoid These Processed, Refined, Harmful Foods:

Once you realize the harm caused to your body by unhealthy refined, chemicalized, deficient foods, you'll want to eliminate "killer" foods:

- **Refined sugar / artificial sweeteners** (toxic aspartame) or their products such as jams, jellies, preserves, marmalades, yogurts, ice cream, sherbets, Jello, cake, candy, cookies, all chewing gum, colas and diet drinks, pies, pastries, and all sugared fruit juices and fruits canned in sugar syrup. (Health Stores have delicious healthy replacements, such as Stevia, raw honey, 100% maple syrup, and agave nectar, so seek and buy the best).

- **White flour products** such as white bread, wheat-white bread, enriched flours, rye bread that has white flour in it, dumplings, biscuits, buns, gravy, pasta, pancakes, waffles, soda crackers, pizza, ravioli, pies, pastries, cakes, cookies, prepared and commercial puddings and ready-mix bakery products. Most are made with dangerous (oxy-cholesterol) powdered milk and powdered eggs. (Health Stores have a variety of 100% non-GMO whole grain organic products, breads, chips, crackers, pastas, desserts).

- **Salted foods,** such as pretzels, corn chips, potato chips, crackers and nuts.

- **Refined white rice** and pearl barley. • **Fried fast foods.** • **Indian ghee.**

- **Refined dry processed cereals** that are sugared, such as cornflakes, etc.

- **Foods that contain Olestra,** palm and cottonseed oil.

- **Peanuts and peanut butter** that contain hydrogenated, hardened oils and any peanuts with mold and all molds that can cause allergies.

- **Margarine** – combines heart-deadly trans-fatty acids and saturated fats.

- **Saturated fats and hydrogenated oils** – enemies that clog the arteries.

- **Coffee, soft drinks, teas, alcohol, sugared juices** – even if decaffeinated.

- **Fresh pork / products.** • **Fried, fatty, greasy meats.** • **Irradiated GMO foods.**

- **Smoked meats,** such as ham, bacon, sausage and all smoked fish.

- **Luncheon meats,** hot dogs, salami, bologna, corned beef, pastrami and packaged meats containing dangerous sodium nitrate or nitrite.

- **Dried fruits** containing sulphur dioxide – a toxic preservative.

- **Chickens, turkeys and meats injected with hormones** or fed with commercial feed containing any drugs or toxins.

- **Canned soups** – read labels for sugar, salt, starch, flour and preservatives.

- **Foods containing preservatives, additives,** benzoate of soda, salt, sugar, cream of tartar, drugs, irradiated and genetically engineered foods.

- **Day-old cooked vegetables,** potatoes and pre-mixed, wilted lifeless salads.

- **All commercial vinegars:** pasteurized, filtered, distilled, white, malt and synthetic vinegars are dead vinegars! (We use only organic raw, unfiltered apple cider vinegar with the "Mother Enzyme" as used in olden times.)

144

Please follow The Bragg Healthy Lifestyle to provide the basic, healthy nourishment to maintain your precious health.

Allergies & Dr. Coca's Pulse Test

Almost every known food may cause some allergic reaction at times. Thus, foods used in elimination diets may cause allergic reactions in some individuals. Some are listed among the *Most Common Food Allergies (see below)*. Since reaction to these foods is generally low, they are widely used in making test diets. By keeping a food journal and tracking your pulse rate after meals you will soon know your problem foods. Allergic foods cause pulse to then go up. *(Take base pulse, for 1 minute, before meals, then 30 minutes after meals, and also before bed. If it increases 8-10 beats per minute – check foods for allergies.)*

If your body has a reaction after eating some particular food, especially if it happens each time you eat that food, you may have an allergy. Some allergic reactions are: wheezing, sneezing, stuffy nose, nasal drip or mucus, dark circles, eye watering or bags under your eyes, headaches, feeling light-headed or dizzy, fast heart beat, stomach or chest pains, diarrhea, extreme thirst, breaking out in a rash, swelling of extremities or stomach bloating. Do read Dr. Arthur Coca's book, *The Pulse Test*.

If you know what you're allergic to, you are lucky; if you don't, you had better find out as fast as possible and eliminate all irritating foods from your diet. To re-evaluate your daily life and have a health guide to your future, start a daily journal *(keep a notebook – enlarge and copy form on next page)* of foods eaten, your pulse rate before and after meals and your reactions, moods, energy levels, weight, elimination and sleep patterns. You will discover the foods and situations causing problems. By charting your diet you will be amazed at the effects of eating certain foods. We have kept daily journals for years.

145

If you are hypersensitive to certain foods, omit them from your diet! There are hundreds of allergies and of course it's impossible here to take up each one. Many have allergies to milk, wheat, or some are allergic to all grains. Visit web: *FoodAllergy.org*. Your daily journal will help you discover and accurately pinpoint the foods and situations causing you problems. Start your journal today!

Most Common Food Allergies

- **DAIRY:** Butter, Cheese, Cottage Cheese, Ice Cream, Milk, Yogurt, etc.
- **CEREALS & GRAINS:** Wheat, Corn, Buckwheat, Oats, Rye
- **EGGS:** Cakes, Custards, Dressings, Mayonnaise, Noodles
- **FISH:** Shellfish, Crabs, Lobster, Shrimp, Shad Roe
- **MEATS:** Bacon, Beef, Chicken, Pork, Sausage, Veal, Smoked Products
- **FRUITS:** Citrus Fruits, Melons, Strawberries
- **NUTS:** Peanuts, Pecans, Walnuts, chemically dried preserved nuts
- **MISCELLANEOUS:** Chocolate, Cocoa, Coffee, Black & Green (caffeine) Teas, Palm & Cottonseed Oils, MSG & Salt. Allergic reactions often caused by toxic pesticides, sprays, etc. on salad greens, vegetables & fruits, etc.

MY DAILY HEALTH JOURNAL

Today is:___/___/___

> *I have said my morning resolve and am ready to practice faithfully The Bragg Healthy Lifestyle today and every day.*

Yesterday I went to bed at:　　　Today I arose at:　　　Weight:

Today I practiced the No-Heavy Breakfast or No-Breakfast Plan: ☐ yes ☐ no

- For Breakfast I drank:　　　　　　　　　　　　Time:

  For Breakfast I ate:

  　　　　　　　　　　　　　　　　　　　　　　Time:

  Supplements:

- For Lunch I ate:　　　　　　　　　　　　　　Time:

  Supplements:

- For Dinner I ate:　　　　　　　　　　　　　　Time:

  Supplements:

- ____ Glasses of Water I Drank during the Day, including ACV Drinks

  List Snacks – Kind and When:

_____

- I took part in these physical activities (walking, gym, etc.) today:

_____

Grade each on scale of 1 to 10 (desired optimum health is 10).
- I rate my day for the following categories:

Previous Night's Sleep:	Stress/Anxiety:
Energy Level:	Elimination:
Physical Activity, Exercise:	Health:
Peacefulness:	Accomplishments:
Happiness:	Self-Esteem:

_____

- General Comments, Reactions and any To-Do List:

Chapter 16

Don't Overeat – It's Harmful To Your Health to Overeat! Eat to Live – Don't Live to Eat

Second after second, minute after minute, hour after hour, day after day our faithful, loyal heart is working to keep us all alive. In both our waking hours and during our sleep, our heart takes only a sixth of a second to rest between beats. The hardest work the heart has to do is right after an individual has eaten! The bigger the meal, the more work your miracle heart has to do in pumping vast quantities of blood into the working digestive tract.

> *Overeating puts more strain on the heart than any other one thing! You should make it a habit to always get up from the table feeling that you could eat a little more!*

Studies done by the Centers for Disease Control and Prevention, found that upwards of 68% of U.S. adults are overweight or obese and the rate is climbing yearly, it's a global epidemic! Obesity is defined when a person's weight (body mass) is over 30% of their ideal body weight. This leads to high triglyceride levels that cause diabetes and cardiovascular disease!

Remember, exercise is a major key factor in lowering your weight and helping keep the heart healthy and fit. Fact: only 20% of Americans exercise one hour weekly, yet they spend over 20 hours watching TV and online weekly.

Childhood obesity rates remain high. Overall, obesity among our nation's young people, ages 2-19 years is currently almost at 20%. More than 40% of adults in U.S. are obese. Overweight children and adults are at high risks for adult on-set heart disease, stroke and type 2 diabetes! Teach your children healthy eating habits by being a healthy, trim, fit example for them!

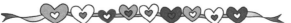

Everything in excess is opposed by Nature!
– Hippocrates, the Father of Medicine, 400 B.C.

It's Proven – Light Eaters Live Longer

My father's research and interviews with people who remained vigorous at ages over 100 years revealed that they ate sparingly, never over-ate and chewed thoroughly! Their diets were well-balanced with simple, natural foods. Scientific tests made on controlled animal feeding have also proven that light eaters live longer and in better health.

Always give thanks first, (millions are starving), then chew food slowly and thoroughly (your stomach has no teeth)! Never eat in a hurry! Food bolted down causes trouble and overworks the stomach and heart! Eating fast produces gas pressure on the heart and can cause a heart attack. If you don't have time to eat correctly, skip that meal! Fasting (pages 163-170), shows skipping a meal is good habit to develop when needed.

Breakfast Should Be An Occasional Meal

Mornings we have our *Energy Smoothie* (page 150) and rare mornings we have organic whole grain cereal, oatmeal or cornmeal, sliced banana or fruit over cereal, with some honey and rice or almond milk.

A rich food source of vitamin E is cornmeal mush, made with organic stoneground yellow cornmeal (not the refined, dead, toxic GMO, degerminated variety found in supermarkets). On next page is the *Bragg family's favorite cornmeal recipe*, plus a chart (page 219) for making sure you get vitamin E from these healthy foods you will enjoy!

148

Maintain Normal Weight by Controlling Your Food Intake

- Swap dinner plates for salad plates, which are usually 2" smaller. You could eat as much as 30% less food. Portion sizes have grown and belly bulge is a result.
- Help with weight loss – order a kid's meal or kid-size portion when dining out.
- Ask for salad dressing on the side. Dip fork in dressing before diving into each bite of salad. It tastes great and you will eat less.
- Order an appetizer instead of an entrée. Have it delivered with everyone's dinner.
- Grocery shop when you are full. Plan a healthy snack before you go and stick to your list to avoid extra food temptations! You will save money too!
- Increase fiber – it's good for your heart and helps promote good elimination. Try these high-fiber foods: apples, raspberries, pears, black beans and broccoli.
- Burn calories in everyday routines. Get off bus one stop earlier. Walk an extra lap around mall. At work, use restroom on floor above you. Tidy your house daily.
- Be active! Walk, exercise, stretch, and dance around when dinner is cooking.

Patricia's Delicious Organic Cornmeal Mush

1 cup organic yellow cornmeal (coarse ground best)
2 1/2 cups distilled water   2 Tbsp raisins or prunes (optional)

Moisten cornmeal with 1/2 cup purified/distilled water. Boil remaining (2 cups) of water, then slowly add moistened cornmeal and raisins. When evenly thickened, turn heat to low and cook for 10-15 minutes. Serve hot, then top with honey, blackstrap molasses or 100% maple syrup, if desired (diabetics use Stevia). Top with sliced bananas or organic fresh fruit and try some almond or rice milk.

NOTE: If you are serving to one or two people, there might be some mush left. Pour it into a flat pan, let it cool, and store in refrigerator. For breakfast – or even a main meal – slice and dip in egg batter and roll in wheat germ. Lightly heat in organic olive oil and serve plain, hot, and top with honey, blackstrap molasses or maple syrup.

Tofu Tasty Scramble

2 cups firm tofu, crumble
2 tsps organic olive oil
1/8 tsp ground cumin
1/4 tsp fresh garlic or powder

2 green onions, chop
tomatoes, diced (optional)
dash of coconut aminos
dash of Italian Seasoning

149

In a wok, lightly sauté green onions in olive oil for 3 minutes, then add remaining ingredients (tomatoes or any fresh grated vegetables desired – keep stirring) cook 5-10 minutes longer. Tasty for breakfast or lunch. Serves 2 to 4.

Tofu Whole Grain French Toast

1/2 lb tofu (soft)
1/4 tsp nutmeg

1/3 tsp cinnamon powder
1 Tbsp honey

Whole grain
bread slices

Blend tofu with enough water (distilled) to make a slightly runny batter. Dip the whole grain bread slices in batter, then lightly sauté until brown in olive oil or butter. Turn over, cook other side. Serve hot with honey or pure maple syrup. Serves 2. *For variety, we often like to have an occasional breakfast of steel-cut organic oats, cooked with raisins, prunes or sliced sun-dried apricots, topped with sliced bananas and 100% maple syrup. Yummy!*

Add an ounce of love to everything you do.

HEALTHY BEVERAGES
Fresh Juices, Herb Teas & Energy Drinks

These freshly squeezed organic vegetable and fruit juices are important to *The Bragg Healthy Lifestyle*. It's not wise to drink beverages with your main meals, as it dilutes the digestive juices. But it's great during the day to have a glass of freshly squeezed orange juice, grapefruit juice, vegetable juice, raw, organic apple cider vinegar drink (see below), or herbal tea – these are all ideal pick-me-up beverages.

Apple Cider Vinegar Drink – Mix 1-2 tsps. raw, organic apple cider vinegar (with the 'Mother' enzyme) and (optional) to taste raw honey or pure maple syrup *(if diabetic, to sweeten use 2 stevia drops)* in 8 oz. of distilled or purified water. Take glass upon arising, an hour before lunch and dinner.

Delicious Hot or Cold Cider Drink – Add 2-3 cinnamon sticks and 4 cloves to water and boil. Steep 20 minutes or more. Before serving add raw organic apple cider vinegar and sweetener to taste.

Bragg's Favorite Juice Drink – This drink consists of all raw vegetables *(remember organic is best)* which we prepare in our juicer / blender: carrots, celery, cucumber, beets, cabbage, tomatoes, watercress, kale, parsley, or any vegetable combination you prefer. The great purifier, garlic we enjoy, but it's optional.

Bragg's Favorite Healthy Energy Smoothie – After morning stretch and exercises we often enjoy drink below instead of fruit. It's a delicious and powerfully nutritious meal anytime: lunch, dinner or in a thermos at work, school, the gym or hiking. You can freeze for popsicles too.

Bragg's Favorite Healthy Energy Smoothie

Prepare the following in a blender, add frozen juice cubes if desired colder; Choice of: freshly squeezed orange or grapefruit juice; carrot and greens juice; unsweetened pineapple juice; or 1 ^{1}/2 - 2 cups purified or distilled water with:

2 tsps spirulina or green powder
^{1}/3 tsp nutritional yeast
2 dates or prunes-pitted
1 "Emergen-C" Vitamin C packet
1 tsp protein powder (optional)

1-2 bananas or fresh fruit
1-2 tsps almond or nut butter
1 tsp flaxseed oil or grind seeds
1 tsp raw honey (optional)
^{1}/2 tsp lecithin granules

Optional: 4-6 apricots (sun-dried,) soak in jar overnight in purified distilled water or unsweetened pineapple juice. We soak enough to last for several days. Keep refrigerated. In summer you can add organic fresh fruit: peaches, papaya, blueberries, strawberries, all berries, apricots, instead of banana. In winter, add apples, kiwi, oranges, tangelos, persimmons or pears, and if fresh is unavailable, try sugar-free, frozen organic fruits. Serves 1 to 2.

Patricia's Delicious Health Popcorn

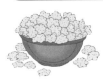

Use freshly popped organic popcorn (use air popper). Drizzle organic olive oil, melted coconut oil or salt-free butter over popcorn. Sprinkle with good quality nutritional yeast for amazing flavor. For a variety try a pinch of cayenne pepper, mustard powder or fresh crushed garlic to oil mixture. Serve instead of breads!

Nutrition directly affects growth, development, reproduction, well-being of an individual's physical and mental condition. Health depends upon nutrition more than on any other single factor. – Dr. William H. Sebrell, Jr.

Lentil & Brown Rice Casserole, Burgers or Soup
Paul Bragg and Jack LaLanne's Favorite Recipe

16 oz pkg organic lentils, uncooked   4 garlic cloves, chop
1 cup brown organic rice, uncooked   2 onions, chop
5 cups, distilled / purified water   2 tsps organic coconut aminos
4-6 carrots, chop $^1/_2$" rounds   1 tsp salt-free all-purpose seasoning
3 celery stalks, chop   2 tsps organic extra-virgin olive oil
1 cup diced fresh or canned tomatoes (salt-free)

Wash and drain lentils and rice. Place grains in large stainless steel pot. Add water, bring to boil, reduce heat and simmer 30 minutes. Now add vegetables and seasonings and cook on low heat until tender. Last five minutes add fresh or canned (salt-free) tomatoes. For delicious garnish, add minced parsley. **For Burgers mash. For Soup, add more water in cooking grains.** Serves 4 to 6.

Patricia's Raw Organic Vegetable Health Salad

2 stalks celery, chop $^1/_2$ cup red cabbage, chop
1 bell pepper & seeds, dice $^1/_2$ cup alfalfa, mung or sunflower sprouts
$^1/_2$ cucumber, slice   2 spring onions & green tops, chop
2 carrots, grate   1 turnip, grate
1 raw beet, grate   1 avocado (ripe)
1 cup green cabbage, chop   3 tomatoes, medium size

For variety add organic raw zucchini, peas, mushrooms, broccoli, cauliflower, (try black olives and pasta). Chop, slice or grate vegetables fine to medium for variety in size. Mix vegetables & serve on bed of lettuce, spinach, chopped kale or cabbage. Dice avocado and tomato and serve on side as a dressing. Serve choice of fresh squeezed lemon, orange or dressing separately. Chill salad plates before serving. **It's best to always eat salad first before hot dishes.** Serves 3 to 5.

(151)

Patricia's Health Salad Dressing

$^1/_2$ cup raw organic apple cider vinegar $^1/_2$ tsp organic coconut aminos
1-2 tsps organic raw honey   1-2 cloves garlic, minced
$^1/_3$ cup organic extra-virgin olive oil, or blend with safflower, sesame or flax oil
1 Tbsp fresh herbs, minced (to taste)

Blend ingredients in blender or jar. Refrigerate in covered jar.

For delicious Herbal Vinegar: In quart jar add $^1/_3$ cup tightly packed, crushed fresh sweet basil, tarragon, dill, oregano, or any fresh herbs desired, combined or singly (if dried herbs, use 1-2 tsps herbs). Now cover to top with raw, organic apple cider vinegar and store two weeks in warm place, and then strain and refrigerate.

Honey – Chia or Celery Seed Vinaigrette

$^1/_4$ tsp dry mustard   1 cup organic apple cider vinegar
$^1/_4$ tsp organic coconut aminos $^1/_2$ cup organic extra-virgin olive oil
$^1/_4$ tsp paprika or to taste $^1/_2$ small onion, minced
1-2 Tbsps honey $^1/_3$ tsp chia or celery seed (or vary to taste)

Blend ingredients in blender or jar. Refrigerate in covered jar.

Studies show both beta carotene and vitamin C, abundantly found in fruits and vegetables, play vital roles in preventing heart disease and cancers.

Food and Product Summary

Today, U.S. foods are highly processed or refined, robbing them of essential nutrients, vitamins, minerals and enzymes. Many also contain harmful, toxic and dangerous chemicals. The research findings and experience of top nutritionists, physicians and dentists have led to the discovery that devitalized foods are a major cause of poor health, illness, cancer and premature death! The enormous increase in the last 70 years of degenerative diseases such as heart disease, arthritis and dental decay substantiate this belief. Scientific research has shown that most of these afflictions can be prevented and that others, once established, can be arrested or even reversed through nutritional methods!

Enjoy Super Health with Natural Foods

1. **RAW FOODS:** Fresh fruits and raw vegetables organically grown are always best! Enjoy nutritious variety garden salads with raw vegetables, sprouts, raw nuts and seeds.

2. **VEGETABLES and PROTEINS:**

   a. Legumes, lentils, brown rice, and all beans.
   b. Nuts and seeds, raw and unsalted.
   c. We prefer healthier vegetarian proteins. If you must have animal protein, then be sure it's hormone–free, and organically fed and no more than 1 or 2 times a week!
   d. Dairy products – fertile range-free eggs (*not over 4 weekly*), unprocessed hard cheese and feta goat's cheese. We choose not to use dairy products. Try the healthier non-dairy oat, rice, and nut-almond milks and tofu cheeses, delicious almond yogurt and rice ice cream.

3. **FRUITS and VEGETABLES:** Organically grown is always best, grown without use of poisonous sprays and toxic chemical fertilizers. Urge markets to stock organic produce! Steam, bake, sauté and stir-fry vegetables as short a time as possible to retain best nutritional content, flavor and use raw veggies in salads, sandwiches, etc. Also enjoy fresh juices.

4. **100% WHOLE GRAIN CEREALS, BREADS and FLOURS:** They contain important B-Complex vitamins, vitamin E, minerals, fiber and the important unsaturated fatty acids.

5. **COLD or EXPELLER-PRESSED VEGETABLE OILS:** organic extra virgin olive oil (is best), sunflower, and flax and sesame oils are excellent sources of healthy, essential, unsaturated fatty acids. We still use oils sparingly.

Bragg Healthy Lifestyle Eating Habits

You need to learn not only what to leave out of your diet, but also, as importantly, what you should put into it. You will find that you can nourish your body without sacrificing meal-time enjoyment once you understand the basic health principles of proper nourishment. This knowledge will show you the elements your body needs to build, develop and live healthily as it was meant to do naturally. Healthy foods: vegetables, fruits, grains, nuts and beans, are packed with vital nutrients.

The first step, of course, is to *get into the habit of eating for health!* Although the instinctive sense of food selection has been submerged with all the advertising of popular fast, junk foods. Like any other ability or skill, a healthy lifestyle must be kept constantly in practice or its powers will deteriorate. Only by exercising this natural health instinct and desire can we revive, strengthen and protect our precious health.

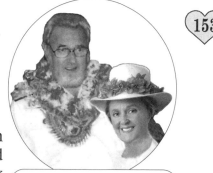

Dr. Koop & Patricia

Hawaii Health Conference

Bad Nutrition – #1 Cause of Sickness

"Diet-related diseases account for 68% of all deaths."
– Dr. C. Everett Koop

(153)

America's former Surgeon General and our friend, said this in his famous landmark report on Nutrition and Health in America. People don't die of infectious conditions as such, but of malnutrition that allows the germs to get a foothold in sickly bodies. Also, bad nutrition is often the cause of non-infectious degenerative conditions. When the body has its full nutrition quota of vitamins and minerals, including potassium, it's almost impossible for germs to get a foothold in a healthy, powerful bloodstream and tissues!

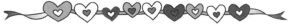

Former U.S. Surgeon General, Dr. C. Everett Koop said –
"Paul Bragg did more for the Health of America than any one person I know of."

Proper Nutrition for Rejuvenation & Fitness

Degenerative diseases stem from breakdowns within the body, not attacks from outside, although the latter may occur secondarily as a result of weakened defenses. Since degenerative diseases arise within our bodies because of some lack of a vital element or substances, our safest course is to reinforce our defenses with those nutrients which will build our powers of resistance. ***Your body is like a fortress.*** Although people may look alike on the *outside, the inside* determines their strengths and weaknesses. Let's build our inner strength so we will be impervious to all deadly enemies of the body!

Don't Clog Arteries with Unhealthy Stimulants & Bad Foods

As poisons accumulate in your body, it becomes impossible to have smooth, flexible arteries through which oxygen-enriched blood can flow freely. The toxins and chemicals from unhealthy foods, saturated fats and caffeinated teas, coffee and colas, leave a poisonous residue on the arteries. Not only do these fats and poisons clog your arteries, but coffee, teas, cola, and alcohol drinks are also unhealthy stimulants to the heart as tobacco smoking is. The heart has a natural rhythm which it can maintain indefinitely under most normal conditions. When you use these harsh stimulants, you actually whip and beat your heart into unnatural activity causing it to be overworked and overstressed.

SAD FACTS: Many people go throughout life committing partial suicide – destroying their health, heart, youth, beauty, talents, energies and creative qualities. Indeed, to learn how to be good to oneself is often more difficult than to learn how to be good to others. – Paul C. Bragg, N.D., Ph.D.

BEING OVERWEIGHT CAN AFFECT YOUR EMOTIONS: Study found that being overweight is associated with specific changes in a part of the brain that is crucial to memory formation and emotions. The Bragg Healthy Lifestyle helps keep you fit and your mind sharp!

Wherever a highly processed food diet becomes the norm, obesity is sure to follow. If you base your diet on primarily packaged, refined processed foods, you are virtually guaranteed to experience weight gain, as they are loaded with white sugar, fructose and refined grains, all of which will pack on unnecessary pounds and make it more difficult to get excess weight off. – Mercola.com

Beware of "Killer" Foods

If drink can kill – so can food! Don't dig your grave with your knife and fork! To have a heart that is fit, your blood chemistry must be healthy and balanced. The 5 to 6 quarts of blood in your body must have all of the *60 nutrients that build and maintain a powerful, fit heart.*

Years ago people did not need to know what to leave out of their diet. That was because the only foods that they had to eat were those produced by Mother Nature. These foods were not robbed of their natural elements like today's foods that are processed and preserved and embalmed by the greedy food industry to stay fresh!

No One Need Suffer Heartburn

If the way to a person's heart is through their stomach, then heartburn (*acid indigestion*) is the end of the romance! Heartburn is a much misunderstood condition that has been written about since Roman times. *First*, it has little to do with the heart. *Second*, it has little to do with spicy or acidic foods. It is caused when the stomach's contents back up into the lower throat (the esophagus). These powerful stomach acids, which are stronger and more acidic than even the spiciest of foods, burn the sensitive walls lining the esophagus.

Reduce Your Acid Reflux and Heartburn

It is vitally important that you don't join the millions of Americans who regularly take a variety of antacids, seltzers, etc. These over-the-counter medications neutralize stomach acids which only further throws off a digestive process already out of balance. You must reduce the amount of fat in your diet because fatty foods cause stomach acids to back up into the esophagus. Also, don't dilute your precious digestive juices by drinking water, juices and herbal teas with your meals. Make it a habit to enjoy beverages between (not during) meals.

To decrease your acid reflux: Avoid eating large meals. Also, avoid excessive alcohol intake, coffee, chocolate, chewing gum, carbonated beverages, citrus juice and raw onions. Elevating the head of your bed may reduce your reflux symptoms and eating too close to bedtime may worsen acid reflux symptoms at night.

When it comes to good digestion, you must practice good posture – sit up tall and straight, lifting up your chest with shoulders slightly back. This will keep your esophagus, stomach and intestines properly aligned and will not crowd your vital organs. Most importantly remember your stomach has no teeth! You must chew each mouthful of food slowly and thoroughly to a pulp that slides down easily! This helps insure a painless, healthy digestion and absorption of more nutrients and energy from your food. – *Mercola.com*

The Deadly Truth About Refined Salt

For centuries, the expression *the salt of the earth* has been used as a catch-all phrase to describe something as good and essential. Yet nothing could be more wrong. That *harmless* product that you shake on top of your food every day may actually bury you way before your time!

Consider these startling facts on salt:

1. ***Refined salt is not a food!*** There is no more justification for its culinary use than there is for potassium chloride, calcium chloride, barium chloride or any other harmful chemical that is used as a food seasoning.

2. ***Salt cannot be digested, assimilated or utilized by the body.*** Salt has no nutritional value! It has no vitamins! No organic minerals! No nutrients of any kind! Instead, it is positively harmful and can cause trouble in the kidneys, bladder, heart, arteries, veins, blood vessels and cause high blood pressure. Salt may waterlog tissues, causing water retention in the body.

3. ***Salt may act as a heart poison.*** It also increases the irritability of the nervous system and the body.

4. ***Salt robs calcium from the body*** and attacks the mucus lining throughout the gastrointestinal tract.

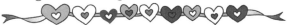

Chewing foods slowly has benefits. Chewing slowly paves the way for better digestion. It helps you eat less. More of the nutrients from your food will be absorbed by your body. It helps you maintain a healthy body weight. Allows you to feel less stress. It's a good exercise for self-discipline. You will experience the taste of your food. Reduces heartburn and indigestion.

What a person eats and drinks becomes his own body chemistry. – Paul C. Bragg

The Myth of the "Salt Lick"

Is a low-salt diet a nutritionally deficient diet? Don't we need plenty of salt in our diets to keep us in top physical condition? This is a popular notion, but is it true? People will tell you that animals will travel for miles to visit so-called *salt licks*. My father investigated the salt licks where wild forest animals congregated for miles around to lick the soil. The one chemical property all of these sites commonly known as *salt licks* had in common was a *complete absence of sodium chloride (common salt)!* There was absolutely no organic or inorganic sodium at the salt licks! *But these soils had an abundance of organic minerals and nutrients which the wise animals naturally craved.*

Salt Affects Your Blood Pressure & Weight

What causes high blood pressure? Medical Science recognizes many causes: diet, obesity, stress, toxic substances such as food additives, insecticide sprays, cigarettes and gasoline fumes, etc. and side effects of drugs and industrial toxins are all suspect! What can you do to protect yourself from these injurious agents? You would do well to exclude as many of these harmful factors from your environment and life as soon as possible!

 However, there is one cause of high blood pressure which can be easily avoided. *Sodium chloride (common table salt) is the major cause of high blood pressure!* Up to now, we have been talking about causing high blood pressure in the *normal* person. But how about the effects of salt on those millions suffering from our country's most prevalent and preventable ailment – excess weight? This is a prime area for research because obesity is known to be frequently accompanied by high blood pressure. Medical researchers proclaim a link between high blood pressure and salt intake in obesity!

The American Heart Association says that daily sodium intake should be less than 2,400 milligrams per day, which is about 1 1/4 teaspoons of sodium chloride (table salt – inorganic sodium). We recommend using NO table salt. Throwing away the salt shaker is a positive step towards living The Bragg Healthy Lifestyle! Get your natural organic sodium from natural healthy foods.

Refined Salt is Not Essential to Life

It is frequently claimed that salt is essential for life. However, there is no scientific basis to this belief. The truth is that entire primitive populations today use absolutely no salt and have never used it (most have no heart disease, arthritis, cancer, etc.). If salt were essential to life, these people would have disappeared long ago.

Break the Deadly Salt Habit – Start Now!

In our expeditions the world over we have met many primitive tribes in the tropics that use no salt. And while they are not bothered by the heat, salt-eating white people invariably complain about the hot weather. This seems to indicate that some commercial motive lies behind the *eat more salt in hot weather* campaign.

People undoubtedly would not add inorganic salt to their food if they were never taught to do so in the first place. ***The taste for salt is an acquired one.*** The craving for salt ceases a short time after it is eliminated from the diet. It is only during the first few weeks after the use of table salt is discontinued that it is really missed. After the initial period of abstinence there is little difficulty. In fact, many of our health students who have broken the deadly salt habit write us to say that now they cannot stand salted foods! When someone serves them salted foods, it gives them an abnormal thirst for liquids!! Their body wants to wash out the salt!

158

The typical American eats 3 times more sodium than the maximum recommended daily intake of 2,400 mgs. This can lead to kidney failure, heart attacks and strokes.

It's a little known fact that about 80% of the sodium we eat comes not from salt we add at the table or during cooking, but comes from salt in many packaged and processed foods (junk foods), as well as restaurant and take-out meals.
– Tufts University Nutrition Letter

According to studies most Americans consume "alarming" amounts of salt that increase the risk of high blood pressure, a major cause of heart disease and strokes. Stick to fresh organic fruits and vegetables and follow The Bragg Healthy Lifestyle.

What Table Salt Does to Your Stomach

An important objection to table salt is the fact that *Salt interferes with the normal digestion of food.* Pepsin, an enzyme found in hydrochloric acid in the stomach, is essential for digestion of proteins. Only 50% as much pepsin is secreted as would otherwise be the case when salt is used! Obviously, digestion of protein foods will be incomplete or too slow under such conditions. The results are excessive putrefaction of protein, gas, bloating and digestive distress, which effects millions!

Sea Kelp is an Excellent Salt Substitute It's a Tasty, Healthy, Organic Sodium

Many outstanding heart specialists heartily endorse a no-salt diet! There are some excellent seasoning substitutes available to satisfy an acquired craving for salt. We use sea kelp, herbs, garlic, and vegetable seasonings. In our opinion, sea kelp is an ideal salt substitute. It gives all foods – salads, vegetables, etc. – a tangy taste. Sea kelp health benefits include: superior nutritional value; detoxification; improved digestive health; contains rare antioxidants; good source of vitamin K; high in trace minerals; and lowers cholesterol. Sea kelp seasonings or granules are rich in iodine for good thyroid health. Fresh or powdered garlic and lemon juice are also excellent seasoners to add delicious flavors to foods.

159

The greatest force in the human body is the natural
drive of the body to heal itself – but that force
is not independent of the belief system.
Everything begins with belief. What we believe
is the most powerful option of all.
– Norman Cousins, author, "Anatomy of an Illness"

The desire for salty foods is an acquired taste. Your taste buds can be retrained to appreciate the true, natural flavors of foods.
– Neal Barnard, M.D., author of "Food for Life"

Shake your unhealthy salt habit! Studies show the salt habit raises risk of heart attack, stroke, hypertension, kidney disease and stomach cancer.
– National Academy of Medicine

Natural Foods Have Organic Sodium

Organic sodium is one of 16 minerals that are *required for perfect mineral balance* in the human body. Absorbable sodium is the most plentiful organic mineral found in all fresh fruits and vegetables, *especially beets, celery and green beans*. Be assured when you eat a balanced diet of plant-based natural foods you will receive sufficient organic sodium.

Your Educated Taste Buds will Guide You

After you give up refined salt you will appreciate the natural flavor of foods. Dad was reared when table salt was used plentifully to season nearly all foods. His 260 taste buds were conditioned to the heavy taste of salt. At 16 he was a victim of tuberculosis. His mother took him to a *Natural TB Sanitarium* where they were against salt in the diet, something new to Dad! His health returned miraculously. His sick body was cleansed and healed – nature's way for a miracle recovery.

160

At first, Dad's taste buds rebelled. But no salt was permitted – so he re-educated his taste buds to a saltless diet. Any bad habit is difficult to overcome at first and the salt habit surely had Dad in its clutches, as salt has millions of Americans! But once his taste buds learned the difference, he started to taste and enjoy the real, natural, healthy flavors of food for the first time in his life!

The Body is Self-Cleansing, Self-Healing and Self-Repairing

It's our duty if we want vibrant, glorious health, to do all we can to make the body work efficiently to maintain vital, super health. Not only is a healthy diet necessary, but so are good sleeping habits, outdoor physical activity, full, deep breathing and a serene, peaceful mind! We cannot live by bread alone. We must have spiritual food. Please strive for a perfect healthy balance: physical, mental, emotional and spiritual well-being!

Let food be your medicine, and medicine be your food. – Hippocrates, 400 B.C.

A fool thinks he needs no advice, but a wise man listens to others. – Proverbs 12:15

Olive Oil – Mediterranean's Tasty Heart Treat

Olives have been used for centuries. Not only are they eaten and used on foods and in cooking, but olive oil is used for ointments, body lotion and in many other ways. In 400 B.C. Hippocrates, the Greek physician (the father of medicine) wrote about the great curative properties of olive oil he called the great therapeutic.

The words of Hippocrates still hold true today. In 1994, the *Lyon Diet Heart Study* wanted to find out why the people of the Mediterranean region had much less heart disease than Americans and Northern Europeans. The answer was found in the characteristic diet of the region. Spaniards, Italians, the French and the Greeks share a diet that is much lower in saturated fats than the diet of those regions with high rates of heart disease. The dietary fat of the Mediterranean residents is primarily olive oil.

The *Lyon Diet Heart Study* and other European research has found that olive oil offers great cardiovascular rewards. After 2 years, people who decreased their fat intake and ate most of the remaining fat in the form of olive oil had a 76% decrease in new heart trouble. The greatest reduction was angina pains and non-fatal heart attacks.

161

Olive oil beneficially influences cardiovascular health by reducing cholesterol levels. It helps protect and strengthen the digestive system by providing the body with *polyphenols* (powerful antioxidant compounds). Don't let this delicious, healthy gift of Mother Nature pass you by! Make organic extra virgin olive oil a part of your healthy heart diet.

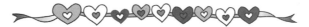

Nutritionist have been studying the Mediterranean diet for the last 20 years and have found that the residents have a very low incidence of heart disease. With the recent discovery of "good" cholesterol (HDL), scientists have begun to understand why people from the Mediterranean area have a very healthy cholesterol balance, with their high consumption of olive oil. This is because olive oil helps stimulate body's production of "good" HDL, that helps the body limit the buildup of substances that block arteries, that cause heart disease.
– Martha Rose Shulman, Author of "Mediterranean Light"

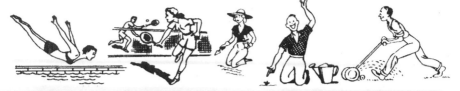

Live The Bragg Healthy Lifestyle
To Enjoy a Lifetime of Super Health!

In a broad sense, *"The Bragg Healthy Lifestyle for the Total Person"* is a combination of physical, mental, emotional, social and spiritual components. The ability of the individual to function effectively in their environment depends on how smoothly these components function as a whole. Of all the qualities that comprise an integrated personality, a totally healthy, fit body is one of the most desirable . . . so start today on your goals for more health, happiness and peace in your life!

A person is said to be totally physically fit if they function as a total personality with efficiency and without pain or discomfort. This is to have a painless, tireless, and ageless body. You possess sufficient muscular strength and endurance to maintain a healthy posture. You can successfully carry on the duties imposed by life and the environment, and meet any emergencies satisfactorily and have enough energy for recreation and social obligations after the "work day" has ended. You possess the body power and Vital Force to recover rapidly from fatigue, and the stress of daily living without the aid of stimulants, drugs or alcohol. You can enjoy recharging sleep at night and awaken fit and alert.

Keeping the body totally healthy and fit is not a job for the uninformed or careless person. It requires an understanding of the body and of a healthy lifestyle and then following that lifestyle for a long, happy life! The purpose of "The Bragg Healthy Lifestyle" is to wake up the possibilities, a rebirth within you, a rejuvenation of your body, mind and spirit for a total balanced body health. It's within your reach, so start today! Daily our hearts and prayers go out to touch your heart and soul with nourishing, caring love for your total health!

With love, your health friends,

Patricia and *Paul C. Bragg*

<p />

Chapter 17

Doctor Fasting

Fasting – the Perfect Heart-Rester

If you are vitally interested in having a strong heart, you must skip 1 or 2 meals a week or even better, fast for one whole day out of 7. What a wonderful rest the hard-working heart receives when you take a day or 2 of total abstinence from all food! Just drink 8-10 glasses distilled water daily (add vinegar to 3, page 150). If you need something warm, have herb tea – mint, alfalfa, anise seed. You may add $1/2$ tsp honey to herb tea or fresh vegetable juices if desired.

A Story of Successful Fasting

We have thousands of letters in our files from health students all over the world, who have had remarkable recoveries with fasting. One of these new students had a serious heart attack at 55 years of age. She was flat on her back in bed for 8 weeks. When she finally got up she was a pitiful sight – pale, haggard and very weak. She was thoroughly discouraged since she had been told she did not have long to live.

Then she got hold of our book *The Miracle of Fasting* and started to fast 1 day each week. Improving after a few months, she fasted for 3 or 4 days each month. Then she went on a 7 day fast. Great cleansing and healing took place in her body because of her fasting and living The Bragg Healthy Lifestyle.

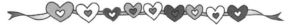

Fasting is the greatest remedy – the physician within!
– *Paracelsus, 15th century physician, established role of chemistry in medicine.*

Along with a weekly 24-hour fast, daily tongue brushing and spoon scraping during oral hygiene (brushing, flossing) is a wise health practice, as your body is continually cleansing from your anus to your tongue. – Patricia Bragg

---

Instead of medicine, fast for a day.
– *Plutarch, Greek Philosopher, 46 A.D.*

Banish All of Your Fears About Fasting!

The average person has a preconceived notion that if they skip a few meals or fast for a few days, dangerous things will happen to their body. Nothing is farther from the truth! My father and I have fasted for as many as 30 days straight – and felt stronger on the 30th day than when the fast started! Caution: We don't advise our students to go on long fasts unless needed and supervised by a health professional.

Nothing will give the body more energy and vitality than fasting. Fasting also strengthens the body's digestive system and heart. Forget your fears! Fasting cleanses the internal body. Try a short fast to demonstrate to yourself the miracles fasting can accomplish in your life!

Cleansing the Heart Pump and Pipes

If our *pipes* and great *pump* are clogged and corroded with debris and toxic poisons we can't be physically fit! Therefore, it's necessary from time to time to give the *pipes* and *pump* of the body a thorough cleansing. This should be done by fasting once every week – for this 1 day will have beneficial effects. It will shake toxins loose from the tissues, stimulate circulation and get rid of foreign matter that has become encrusted in the heart and blood vessels.

Here's our personal fasting program for you: We fast on Mondays. During this time we drink 8 to 10 glasses of distilled water, 3 with apple cider vinegar (page 150). This gives our digestive and elimination systems a complete rest. We then eat on Tuesday. This rest from food takes a great load off of the hard-working heart and digestive system and helps keep the body cleaner and healthier!

You should follow this cleansing program at least one day a week. Then in time you will have enough fortitude to fast for 3 days straight – you will be amazed at the results! If you have any reactions during this cleansing program – such as headaches, excessive gas or feelings of weakness – just remember that this is what we call a *healing crisis*. These symptoms will fade away as the toxins pass out through your elimination system.

Flushing Poisons from Your Body's "Pipes"

While on this *Cleansing Program*, drink at least a half a gallon of distilled (purified) water daily – that is free of toxic chemicals. The night before you start this regime make a **Green Drink:** *take 1 to 2 quarts of distilled water and add to it 2 whole carrots cut into pieces, 3 diced stalks of celery (leaves and all), 1 handful of chopped parsley and 2 beets cut up fine. Soak this mixture overnight. After it has soaked 10 hours or more, strain the vegetable-distilled water and discard the vegetables (great for compost). Use this water, in which the vegetables have been soaked, as part of your drinking water during first day for your cleansing.*

ON ARISING have an apple cider vinegar drink (page 150) an hour later eat an apple and a few sun-dried figs or dates, 1 glass of prune juice (add 1 tsp. mixed oat bran and psyllium).

AT 10 A.M. eat some fresh fruit (oranges, grapefruit, bananas, apples, pears, grapes, etc.) and drink a cup of herbal tea or "green drink" see above for instructions. If you take supplements, do so now.

AT 12 NOON enjoy a tossed green salad of sliced cabbage with grated carrots and beets, chopped green onion, celery, bell pepper, parsley, raw spinach, watercress, tomato and 2 cloves finely chopped garlic. Eat this salad with the salad dressing recipes found on page 151 or any healthy salad dressings. You may also have a lightly cooked vegetable (low in natural sugar) such as string beans, squash or any green leafy vegetables, kale, etc.

AT 3 P.M. eat fresh fruit, such as apples, grapes, pears, bananas or a few dried fruits such as dates, figs and prunes, and a cup of hot distilled water with a squeeze of lemon.

AT 6 P.M. supper, tossed vegetable/green salad as lunch and bowl of lightly steamed greens (kale, mustard or turnip greens, beet tops, spinach) cooked with chopped onions, 2 garlic cloves and before serving add 1 Tbsp. organic olive oil. After meal you may take your evening supplements.

165

Flaxseed Cleanse: Soak 1 Tbsp. of flaxseeds (for 1 hour) in a glass of distilled water, then add a cup of herbal tea and stir. Drink 1 hour after dinner which is the best time or you may substitute a psyllium husk vegetarian capsule.

Blender/Juice Fast – Introduction to Water Fast

Fasting has been rediscovered, through juice fasting, as a simple, easy means of cleansing and restoring health and vitality. To fast (abstain from food) comes from the Old English word *fasten* or *to hold firm.* It's a means to commit oneself to the task of finding inner strength through body, mind and soul cleansing. Throughout history the world's greatest philosophers and sages – including Socrates, Plato, Buddha, Gandhi and Jesus – practiced fasting and preached its benefits!

Juice/Blender Bars are more commonplace and those who believe in the power and effectiveness of juice and water fasting is growing! They say fasting helps balance their lives physically, mentally, spiritually and emotionally. Although we feel a water fast is best, an introductory liquid juice fast can offer people an ideal opportunity to give their intestinal systems a restful, cleansing relief from the high fat, high sugar, high salt and high protein fast foods too many Americans unhealthfully exist on!

Organic, raw, live fruit and vegetable juices can be purchased fresh from Health Stores. You can also prepare these healthy drinks yourself using a good juicer/blender. When juice fasting, it's best to dilute juice with $1/3$ distilled water. The list on the next page gives many delicious combination ideas. With any vegetable and tomato combinations try adding a dash of herbs or on non-fast days, even try some green powder (barley, chlorella, spirulina, etc.) to create a delicious, nutritious, powerful health drink. When using herbs in these drinks, use 1 to 2 fresh leaves or try sea kelp seasoning (see page 159 for more information), which is rich in protein, iodine and is delicious with vegetable juices.

Fasting is an effective and safe method of detoxifying the body – a technique used for centuries for healing. Fast regularly one day a week and help the body cleanse and heal itself to stay well. When a cold or illness is coming on, or even depression – it's best to fast! Bragg Books were my conversion to the healthy way.
– James Balch, M.D. Co-Author of "Prescription for Nutritional Healing"

Wherever you go, no matter what the weather,
always bring your own sunshine. – Anthony J. D'Angelo

Healthy, Delicious Juice / Blender Combinations:

1. *Beet, celery, alfalfa sprouts*
2. *Cabbage, celery and apple*
3. *Cabbage, cucumber, celery, tomato, spinach and basil*
4. *Tomato, carrot and celery*
5. *Carrot, celery, watercress, apple, garlic and wheatgrass*
6. *Grapefruit, orange and lemon*
7. *Beet, parsley, celery, carrot, mustard greens, cabbage, garlic*
8. *Beet, celery, kelp and carrot*
9. *Cucumber, carrot and celery*
10. *Watercress, apple, cucumber, garlic*
11. *Asparagus, carrot and celery*
12. *Carrot, celery, parsley and cabbage, onion, sweet basil*
13. *Carrot, coconut milk and ginger*
14. *Carrot, broccoli, lemon, cayenne*
15. *Carrot, sprouts, kelp, rosemary*
16. *Apple, carrot, radish, ginger*
17. *Apple, pineapple and ginger*
18. *Apple, papaya and grapes*
19. *Papaya, cranberries and apple*
20. *Leafy greens, broccoli, apple*
21. *Grape, apple and blueberries*
22. *Watermelon (alone is best)*

Enjoy Healthy Fiber for Super Health
From UC Berkeley Wellness Letter

These are our suggestions for healthy fiber:

- EAT ALL VARIETIES OF ORGANIC BERRIES, surprisingly good sources of fiber.

- KEEP BEANS HANDY, probably the best fiber sources. Cook dried beans and freeze in portions. Use canned beans for faster meals.

- INSTEAD OF ICEBERG LETTUCE, choose deep green lettuces such as romaine, bib, butter, spinach or cabbage.

- LOOK FOR "100% ORGANIC WHOLE WHEAT" or whole grain breads, when eating bread.

- LOOK FOR WHOLE GRAIN or RICE CEREALS.

- GO FOR BROWN RICE over white rice.

- EAT THE SKIN of the potato, fruits and vegetables.

- SERVE HUMMUS, made from chickpeas, instead of sour-cream with your dip.

- DON'T UNDERESTIMATE NON-GMO ORGANIC CORN, especially popcorn and corn tortillas.

- ADD ORGANIC OAT BRAN & WHEAT-GERM to baked goods.

- SNACK ON ORGANIC SUN-DRIED FRUIT.

- INSTEAD OF DRINKING FRUIT JUICE, eat whole fruit.

Wherever flaxseed becomes a regular food item among the people, there will be better health. – Mahatma Gandhi

Fasting Cleanses, Renews and Rejuvenates

Our bodies have a natural self-cleansing system for maintaining a healthy body and our *river of life* – our blood. It's essential that we keep our entire bodily machinery healthy and in good working condition from head to toe!

Fasting is the best detoxifying method. It's also the most effective and safest way to increase elimination of waste buildups and enhance the body's miraculous self-healing and self-repairing process that keeps you healthy.

If you prepare for a fast by eating a cleansing diet for 1 to 2 days, this can greatly facilitate the cleansing process. Fresh variety salads, fresh vegetables and fruits and their juices, as well as green drinks (alfalfa, barley, chlorophyll, chlorella, spirulina and wheatgrass) stimulate waste elimination. Live, fresh foods and organic fruit and vegetable juices can literally pick up dead matter from your body and carry it away. You can start your liquid fast by following this pre-cleansing diet. Several times yearly we commit to a longer *super* fast. We usually prefer a distilled water fast for 7 to 10 days. This works wonders in keeping us fit, trim and healthy (page 170)!

Daily, even on most days during our fasts, we take 3,000 mg. of mixed Vitamin C "Emergen-C" powder (C concentrate, Acerola, Rose hips and Bioflavonoids) in liquids. This is a potent antioxidant and flushes out deadly free radicals. It also promotes collagen production for new healthy tissues. *Vitamin C is especially important if you are detoxifying from prescription drugs, alcohol or stress overload,* stated by our friend, famous scientist Dr. Linus Pauling.

A moderate, well-planned distilled water fast is our favorite or a diluted fresh juice (35% distilled water) fast can help cleanse your body of excess mucus, old fecal matter, trapped cellular, non-food wastes and can help remove inorganic mineral deposits and sludge from your pipes and joints. Fasting works by self-digestion. During a fast your body intuitively will decompose and burn only the substances and tissues that are damaged, diseased or unneeded, such as abscesses, tumors, excess fat deposits, excess water and congestive wastes. (See benefits page 170.)

Fasting is Your Body's Miracle Cleanser

Even on a short health fast (1-3 days) your body will accelerate elimination from your liver, kidneys, lungs, bloodstream and skin. Sometimes you will experience dramatic changes (a cleansing and healing crisis) as accumulated wastes are expelled! With your first few fasts you may temporarily have headaches, fatigue, body odor, bad breath, a coated tongue, mouth sores and even diarrhea as your body is cleaning house. *Be patient with your body!*

After a fast your body will begin to respond and healthfully rebalance. When you follow The Bragg Healthy Lifestyle, your weekly 24-hour fast removes toxins on a regular basis, so they don't accumulate. Your energy levels will begin to rise – physically, psychologically and mentally. Your creativity will begin to expand. You will feel like a *different person* – which you are – as you're being cleansed, purified and reborn! Fasting is an exciting and wonderful detox cleansing and miracle healing blessing for your body.

169

For Easier Flowing Bowel Movements

It's natural to squat to have bowel movements. It opens up the anal area more directly. When on the toilet, putting feet up 6 to 8 inches on a waste basket or footstool gives the same squatting effect. Now raise arms, stretch hands above head so the transverse colon can empty completely with ease. It's important for you to drink 8 to 10 glasses pure water daily – works miracles! After dinner meal take 1 psyllium husk veg. cap daily or do Flaxseed Cleanse (page 131).

ELIMINATE THE "DRIBBLES" EXERCISE:
To keep bladder and sphincter muscles tight and toned, urinate – stop – urinate – stop, 6 times, twice daily when voiding, especially after age 40. This simple exercise works wonders for both men and women!

There is just one life for each of us: our own. – Euripides

Good elimination is vitally important for your health and longevity!

(BENEFITS FROM THE JOYS OF FASTING)

Fasting renews your faith in yourself, your strength and God's strength.
Fasting is easier than any diet.
Fasting is the quickest way to lose weight.
Fasting is adaptable to a busy life.
Fasting gives the body a physiological rest.
Fasting is used successfully in the treatment of many physical illnesses.
Fasting can yield weight losses of up to 10 pounds or more in the first week.
Fasting lowers and normalizes cholesterol, homocysteine, blood pressure levels.
Fasting improves dietary habits.
Fasting increases pleasure eating healthy foods.
Fasting is a calming experience, often relieving tension and insomnia.
Fasting frequently induces feelings of happy euphoria, a natural high.
Fasting is a miracle rejuvenator, helps in slowing the ageing process.
Fasting is a natural stimulant to rejuvenate the growth hormone levels.
Fasting is an energizer, not a debilitator.
Fasting aids the elimination process.
Fasting often results in a more vigorous happy marital relationship.
Fasting can eliminate smoking, drug and drinking addictions.
Fasting is a regulator, educating the body to consume food only as needed.
Fasting saves precious time spent on marketing, preparing and eating.
Fasting rids the body of toxins, giving it an internal shower and cleansing.
Fasting does not deprive the body of essential nutrients.
Fasting can be used to uncover the sources of food allergies.
Fasting is used effectively in schizophrenia and other mental illness treatment.
Fasting under proper supervision can be tolerated easily up to four weeks.
Fasting does not accumulate appetite; hunger pangs disappear in 1-2 days.

170 Fasting is routine for most of the animal kingdom.
Fasting has been a common practice since the beginning of man's existence.
Fasting is practiced in all religions; the Bible alone has 74 references to fasting.
Fasting under proper conditions is absolutely safe.
Fasting is a blessing – "Fasting As A Way Of Life" – Allan Cott, M.D.
Fasting is not starving, it's nature's cure that God has given us. – Patricia Bragg

Dear Health Friend,

This gentle reminder explains the great benefits from "The Miracle of Fasting" that you will enjoy when starting on your weekly 24-hour Bragg Fasting Program for Super Health! It's a precious time of body-mind-soul cleansing and renewal.

On fast days I drink 8-10 glasses of distilled (our favorite) or purified water, (I add 1-2 tsps. organic, raw apple cider vinegar to three of them). If just starting, you may also try herbal teas or try diluted fresh juices with 1/3 distilled water. Every day, even on fast days, add 1 Tbsp. of psyllium husk powder to liquids once daily. It's an extra cleanser and helps normalize weight, cholesterol and blood pressure and helps promote healthy elimination. Fasting is the oldest, most effective healing method known to man. Fasting offers great miraculous blessings from Mother Nature and our Creator. It begins the self-cleansing of the inner-body workings so we can promote our own self-healing.

My father and I wrote the book "The Miracle of Fasting" to share with you the health miracles it can perform in your life. It's all so worthwhile to do. It's an important part of The Bragg Healthy Lifestyle.

With Love, *Patricia*

Paul Bragg's work on fasting and water is one of the great contributions to The Healing Wisdom and The Natural Health Movement in the world today.
– Gabriel Cousens, M.D., Author "Conscious Eating" and "Spiritual Nutrition"

Chapter 18

Doctor Rest

Sound Sleep is Necessary To Build a Strong Heart

Primitive men and women would arise at daybreak and the early hours of their days were spent in vigorous physical activity. About mid-day they would eat their largest meal and then immediately afterward would lie down to rest or take a nap (just as babies, young children and even animals do). In an hour they would wake up refreshed – ready for the 2nd half of the day. They were active again until sundown, and shortly afterwards go to sleep again. So primitive man was awake about 12 hours and slept about 12 hours.

Modern, civilized man drives himself all day under high-pressure. His day is filled with stresses, strains, worries and cares. A daily nap or *siesta* is unknown to the routine of most people. All day long he takes many stimulants to keep himself going – coffee, tea, alcohol, pills, cigarettes, excessive amounts of sugar, candy, chocolate, ice-cream, etc. – everything to try to keep his poor body up to the constant *go, go – push mode*!

He lives in this hectic, fast driven age and at night he has brilliant lights and action to keep him awake. His amusements and entertainments all begin at night. The night clubs turn on bright lights and loud music. TV, web, videos, radio, parties – everything seems to be geared to stimulate him. Instead of going to bed for much needed sleep he drives himself, chasing happiness and peace of mind.

When he gets sleepy he just takes a pill, and to keep him awake, drinks some strong coffee, then to relax he has some poisonous alcohol. He is constantly straining his nervous system – all of which has a disastrous deadly effect on his circulatory system and his heart!

Think of yourself as a "battery" – you discharge energy and you must recharge yourself with proper food, sleep and constructive emotions.
– Patricia Bragg, Pioneer Health Crusader

The majority of American's nerves are so frazzled and burned-out that it's often impossible for them to get a good night's sleep. As a result, *they consume sleeping pills and tranquilizers* to calm their exhausted nervous systems. It's no wonder that, in addition to the *soaring heart disease rate in the United States*, we have more people with mental disorders than ever before in history. Mental Health facilities are now so over-crowded that they represent one of our society's greatest medical and financial problems today. For more peaceful, calm and healthy nerves read the Bragg book *Building Powerful Nerve Force*.

Sleep is Essential To Life Itself

You cannot have a strong heart, a sound mind and a healthy nervous system if you do not get enough good and sound restful sleep! Sleep is essential to building and maintaining a strong, vital heart. *Sleep is more necessary than food!* Anyone can fast on water for days – or even weeks if necessary – without any serious harm if they are well-nourished before beginning the fast and have a satisfactory food-supply after its conclusion. But no one can *fast* from sleep for a few days without side effects. Man can't endure an entire week of sleeplessness.

In early English history condemned criminals were put to death by depriving them of sleep. This forced sleeplessness, in fact, has been used as a form of torture and execution by some countries and is more feared than corporal punishment. Those subjected to this always died raving maniacs! Sad facts illustrate the necessity of sleep!

Take a Daily "Siesta"

If you want to build a *strong heart* and *nervous system*, take a mid-day nap. Getting an hour's rest in the middle of the day is like having 2 days in 1, when you wake up after your *siesta* you have a stored up great nervous energy reserve. We believe people of Mexico, South America and Europe had a healthy idea when they followed the policy of closing down businesses from noon to 2 pm for lunch and siesta. Rest is important for building a powerful body and heart!

Help me to know the magic of rest, relaxation and the restoring power of sleep.

How Much Sleep Do We Need?

How much sleep do we need? Every individual is different. Some people require more sleep than others! Those often possessing greater vitality and stronger constitutions require less sleep than those of limited vitality and weaker recuperative powers. Those who possess a strong metabolic system and great vitality can store energy during sleep and also recover from the exertions of the preceding day more rapidly. A strong person will be restored more quickly than others. Their system can more rapidly repair the wear and tear of their daily work than that of a weaker individual.

University of Chicago research has found strong signs of *accelerated* ageing in healthy young men after less than a week in which they slept for just four hours per night. Not getting enough sleep can age people prematurely and promote illness! Getting 12 hours of sleep for several nights turned the students back to their right age.

Most people need 7 to 9 hours of sleep nightly. Women and children require a bit more sleep. We feel that 8 hours of sleep per night is important for a strong heart and that 1 to 2 hours of this sleep should be obtained before midnight. A single hour of sleep before midnight is worth 3 hours of sleep. We enjoy 30-60 minute afternoon naps when possible – the siesta habit is great!

Rules for Restful, Recharging Sleep

It's best to *sleep with your head to the north*, so you will be in direct contact with the Earth's vibrations, and on an outside porch or in a room with good cross-ventilation. Weather permitting you can sleep nude or in non-constricting natural (cotton, silk, wool) garments. Sleep with a head cradle pillow so that your neck and spine are aligned and your heart won't have to pump so hard against gravity. Sleeping in a cramped position, on a soft mattress (firm is best) or in a manner that blocks circulation is not conducive to restful sleep. In bed, stretch and spread your body out, then practice slow deep breathing and sleep peacefully.

A study at the College of Holy Cross in Massachusetts found students who got less sleep, got poorer grades! Teens need 8 to 10 hours sleep per night.

Your Mattress is Your Best Sleeping Friend

You should sleep on a firm mattress or place a board under a soft one. This allows the muscles to stretch in natural relaxation and relieves pressure on vital organs.

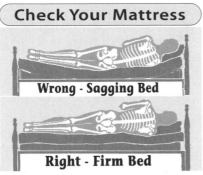

Check Your Mattress

Wrong - Sagging Bed

Right - Firm Bed

The right kind of mattress is important! You should sleep on a firm mattress

When on our world lecture tours, we would often have to move our mattresses onto the floor to be firmer. It seems that some of the world's top hotels put their money into showy lobbies and not into firm mattresses. We often found old, sagging mattresses in many of the homes we visited – but new cars in their garages! Try a miracle foam mattress pad on top of the mattress – it's great. It might take you a few nights to become accustomed to being stretched out flat – but soon your body will thank you with more energy.

174

We traveled all over the world in trains, planes, ships, buses and automobiles and would often use soft foam ear plugs to shut out unnecessary sounds and noises. We feel it's absolutely necessary that we sleep in a place that is quiet! Even though we often do fall asleep when there is noise all about us, the vibratory action of the noise can have a direct effect on the heart, circulation and nervous system.

The Serenity Prayer

Grant me the serenity to accept
  the things I cannot change,
The courage to change the things I can,
And the wisdom to know the difference. ~ *Reinhold Niebuhr*

You are a Miracle – Self-Cleansing, Self-Repairing, Self-Healing –
Please become aware of "YOU" and be thankful for all your
miracle blessings that take place daily! – Paul C. Bragg, N.D., Ph.D.

The electromagnetic radiation from internet routers (Wi-Fi) is weaker than cell phones, but turn off when not using. To be extra safe keep cell phones, computers, laptops and other electronics away from where you sleep. – doctoroz.com

America's National "Sleep Debt"

National Sleep Foundation polls remark that a whopping 69% of American adults have a sleeping problem and 40% are so sleepy during the daytime that their daily activities are interfered with. Few are lucky enough to enjoy 5-6 hours of sound sleep and still perform well at work. Over the past 100 years, we've reduced our average sleep time by 20% and, over the last 25 years, we've added an additional month to our annual work-commute time. Thus, our national *sleep debt* is rising and while our society has changed, our physical bodies and needs have not. Just to get caught up, a full 10 hours of rest is frequently called for!

So, the odds are you aren't getting sufficient sleep. American adults presently average 7 hours nightly. While everyone's sleep needs vary, **Scientific Research Studies indicate we require at least 8 hours of sleep nightly.**

Before Calling it a Night . . .

First make a conscious choice about how you wish to spend the 30 to 45 minutes before bedtime. Avoid a rush to *get things ready for tomorrow* or to catch up on tasks not completed during the day. Slow down your body and mind with an aroma-therapeutic/massage bath and enjoy a soothing lemon balm tea drink before bedtime and a melatonin (1mg.) cap aids sleep, plus fights free radicals.

 175

Try Lemon Balm for a Night So Calm

Lemon Balm, whose scientific name is *melissa officinalis,* is a cooling plant with both nervine and antiseptic qualities. As a member of the *Labiatae* family, which also includes peppermint and spearmint, lemon balm is native to most areas of Europe and has been widely grown worldwide. Flowering between June and October, its lemon-like fragrance is unmistakable.

Research shows that sleep deprivation increases the risk of high blood pressure and heart disease. Sleep deprivation can change the body's secretion of hormones. These changes promote over-eating and alter the body's response to sugar intake – changes that can promote weight gain and increase the risk of developing diabetes. – Newsweek

Like restful chamomile, lemon balm's primary, volatile oils make the plant medicinal. While appearing to be just a simple plant, it delivers a wide range of rather potent cures, ranging from stomach pain to the worst cases of insomnia. Try lemon balm tea before bedtime – miraculous results have been reported and it can be blended with a variety of herbal teas. Also others to try for sound sleep are: *Sleepytime tea*, skullcap, valerian herbal teas, magnesium and calcium supplements and melatonin (1 mg) before bedtime.

Tips for Healthful Sound Sleep

- Avoid stimulants such as caffeine, found in coffee, tea, chocolate, soda, and nicotine, found in cigarettes and other tobacco products.
- Don't drink alcohol to "help" you sleep.
- Exercise regularly, but be finished with your workout routine no sooner than 3 hours prior to bedtime.
- Establish a regular and relaxing bedtime routine; for example, try an aromatherapy bath or a relaxing shower.
- Associate your bed with relaxing, recharging sleep – don't use it for doing work or watching TV.
- If you often suffer from insomnia, don't take naps.

Relief for the Snorer in the House

Now there are choices in treatment for relieving snoring. A simple nasal strip (adhesive band-aid-like device) that helps keep open nose's nasal passages and allows easier airflow during sleep is available at pharmacies, sizes small to large.

The second option is RIPSNORE™. A simple, one-piece device that molds to the shape of your mouth. The device is very flexible when being fitted. It stops snoring or drastically reduces snoring in 98% of people who started using it. The RIPSNORE™ holds the lower jaw slightly forward, moving base of tongue away from back of airway and soft palate - allowing throat to be opened and the snore to be silenced. The device is almost identical to dental ones, but is a lot more affordable. To order on web: *www.RipSnore.com*

Chapter 19

Safer, Non-Invasive Tests & Natural Therapy

Heart Surgery Versus Natural Therapy

Often our Western medical professionals turn first to invasive procedures rather than safer and less expensive non-invasive, healthier alternatives. This is true in both diagnosis and treatment.

A *coronary angiogram* is a diagnostic test that measures blood flow and blockages in the heart. A catheter is inserted into patient's leg artery (through the groin or arm), and threaded up through artery to patient's heart.

A Harvard University medical study reports that invasive heart surgeries have little effect on the long-term survival of most heart patients. Only in the most severe cases did dangerous, invasive operations show significant statistical merit! The study suggested that these types of surgeries could be reduced by 25% or more without endangering the health of heart patients. Rather than using this important study's advice, doctors are increasing expensive heart surgeries at an alarming rate!

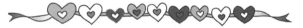

Wise Health Advise from Dr. Dean Ornish: We tend to think of advances in medicine as being a new drug, new surgical technique, new laser, something high-tech and expensive. We often have a hard time believing the simple choices we make each day in our diet and lifestyle can make such a powerful difference in the quality and quantity of our lives, but they most often do. My health program consists of four main parts: exercise, nutrition, stress management, love and support. These promote not only living longer, but living better. – ornish.com.

---

*Whatever occurs in the mind, affects the body and visa versa.
Mind and body cannot be considered independently. When the two are
out of sync, both the emotional and physical stress can erupt.
– Hippocrates, the Father of Medicine, 400 B.C.*

---

*Good health, generated by physical fitness is the logical starting point
for the pursuit of excellence in any field. Physical vitality promotes
mental vitality and thus is essential to executive achievement.
– Dr. Richard E. Dutton, University of Southern Florida*

Safer Minimally Invasive Surgery

Continued advances have brought safer alternatives to open heart surgery techniques. Minimally Invasive Surgery was originally conceived by a Russian Surgeon in the early 1960's. Procedures are now performed through an incision less than $1/3$ the size of a drastic full sternotomy (the former ranges from 9-12 cm long, the latter averages 30 cm). Two types of procedures are being done using this technique: minimally invasive direct coronary artery bypass, or MIDCAB, and minimally invasive valve repair and replacement. MIDCAB is the "beating heart" surgery since the heart doesn't have to be stopped or placed on cardiopulmonary bypass (the heart-lung machine that oxygenates the blood and maintains blood pressure) and surgeons can operate while the heart continues to beat, which is safer for the patient. Due to the reduced incision size, this technique is less traumatic, has shorter recovery time and helps reduce the need for pain-killers.

The Safer Road to Reduce Heart Disease

Dr. Julian Whitaker, one of America's famous heart specialists, became so outraged years ago over unsafe trends that he says, *"I gave up being a surgeon to become a healer."* He founded the renowned Whitaker Wellness Institute in Newport Beach, California, and has the popular health newsletter, *Health and Healing.* A healthy lifestyle like The Bragg Healthy Lifestyle is his alternative to angiograms and surgery.

Dr. Dean Ornish, the Clinical Professor of Medicine, School of Medicine, UCSF, is another world famous doctor-turned-healer. When Ornish's heart patients embraced a healthy, energetic exercise regime and ate nutritious, low-fat foods, their heart conditions began improving within one month! After a year, most patients had virtually no chest pains or heart problems! For 82% of his patients a healthy lifestyle reversed their arterial clogging!

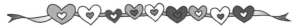

Medical and Hospital Emergency Centers do fast tests to relieve your mind to see if you have had a mild heart attack. It's better to be safe than sorry.

Find the Right Doctor to Protect Your Heart

Safer, less expensive, non-invasive alternatives can bring about greater health. Invasive heart tests and operations can be dangerous, costly and often unnecessary! There are a growing number of doctors that specialize in protecting heart patients from the use of angiograms, bypass surgery and angioplasty. As an alternative they place sonar devices, electronic sensors and microphones, on the outside of the chest. These sensitive tests can often judge heart disease better than procedures which use dangerous, invasive catheters, tubes and needles.

When needed, consult with health physicians and organizations that are dedicated to making the healthcare of your heart a wise, safer job.

Blood Tests Reveal Risks of Heart Disease

It is often said that you're probably not at risk for heart disease if your LDL (Low Density Lipoprotein) level is low (see inside front cover). However, a recent study published in the *American Heart Journal* concluded that almost half of the patients with cardiovascular disease actually had low LDL levels (less than 100mg/dl). This is contrary to standard belief! According to the National Cholesterol Education Program, new risk factors for heart disease include high amounts of small, dense LDL. This type of LDL is dangerous as it can be easily oxidized by free radicals (see page 25-27) and can penetrate into the delicate inner lining of the blood vessel walls to form plaque. In contrast, large LDL do not put you at increased risk. This may sound confusing, but by taking these special tests, you may be able to detect heart disease more efficiently.

Oxygen is one of the primary catalysts for energy and optimal health in the human body!

So this morning begin by eating God's natural foods, drink pure water, think positive thoughts, affirm aloud, take healthy action and tomorrow will be brighter, happier and healthier than you ever dreamed possible!
– Robert Anthony Schuller, former pastor, Crystal Cathedral

Check Out These Important Blood Tests

• **NMR (Nuclear Magnetic Resonance) Lipoprofile:** *LDL Particle Number and LDL Particle Size* are the most important factors in determining if you are at risk for heart disease, according to research (*www.mercola.com*). If you have *MANY LDL Particles that contain LESS cholesterol in each particle, your heart disease risk will be high even if your measured LDL level is low.* (Remember LDL is your "bad" cholesterol). The greater number of cholesterol-containing particles in the blood means more cholesterol is deposited in plaque.

Also *LDL Particles* vary in size. The size difference is crucial. *SMALL LDL Particles are far more destructive than their larger counterparts.* Smaller particles penetrate more effectively into the cellular barrier and enter arterial walls, contributing to atherosclerotic plaque. They also persist longer in the circulation, which allows them to cling to tissues within the walls. Once in the arterial wall, small LDL particles are more prone to oxidation, which stimulates the release of inflammatory and adhesive proteins. All in all small LDL is more likely to contribute to the build-up of plaque within arteries than normal LDL. Small LDL particles triple the likelihood of developing coronary plaque and suffering a heart attack.

The LDL Lipoprofile test reflects the total concentration of cholesterol within the LDL Particles.

Learning is finding out what you already knew.
Doing is demonstrating that you know it!
Teaching is reminding others that they know it
just as well as you! You are all learners,
doers and teachers! – Richard Bach

We are a product of our thoughts – and so is our health! While doctors and medicine have their place, self-healing is the most powerful medicine of all. Accepting the present and placing trust in a higher power frees your energy to focus on improving your life! See problems as challenges of growth, not as a punishment or judgement! Focus on happiness, forgiveness, hope and peace of mind, as well as physical change to ease any problems and situations.

Harvard School of Public Health Study found 84% of those who sought a second opinion after scheduling heart bypass surgery, were told they didn't need it!

- **High-Sensitivity C-Reactive Protein (CRP) Test:** CRP is an independent risk factor for heart disease, a known inflammatory compound that could be damaging to the blood vessel walls, setting you up for plaque formation, inflammation and possible heart attack (see page 48).

- **Homocysteine Test:** Homocysteine is a by-product of your body's metabolism. When high it can increase inflammation of your blood vessel walls (see page 50).

- **Fibrinogen Test:** Fibrinogen is a blood clotting factor, if it is high, you are at risk of forming blood clots that could lead to a heart attack or stroke. A systemic enzyme supplement helps maintain a more normal inflammatory response and helps maintain safe fibrin levels for a more healthy cardiovascular system.*

These specialized tests can give a much better picture of your risk for heart disease. But even if your results from all these tests are within normal ranges, you will still be wise when you choose to follow The Bragg Healthy Lifestyle.

MRI – Non-Invasive Window into the Heart

Doctors use *magnetic resonance imaging* (MRI) as a non-invasive, diagnostic tool to look at soft tissue inside patients without having to invade the body. MRIs use a powerful, but harmless magnetic field that reveal in great detail, the shape and condition of your internal organs. Doctors use this test to diagnose various heart and entire body conditions.

What can a non-invasive MRI procedure tell a doctor about patient's heart and circulatory system? Miracle MRIs identify heart scarring and any other indications of a previous or future heart attack. It can reveal arterial clogging and the presence of any foreign masses in and around heart and body. It detects signs of heart disease, identifies vascular disorders (an enlarged heart) and checks vessel health. **Warning: MRIs cannot be used on people with pacemakers or arterial clips.**

Open your mind, for the doors of wisdom are never shut.
– Benjamin Franklin

---

*This statement has not been evaluated by the Food and Drug Administration. This product is not intended to diagnose, treat, cure or prevent any disease.

Seek These Safer and Healthier Non-Invasive Tests for Heart Disease:

DOPPLER COLOR FLOW IMAGING TEST: This is a safe, non-invasive imaging ultrasound. It shows a clear profile that checks the entire blood vessel system simultaneously. When needed, doctors check for possible blood slow-down and blockages that can cause future heart attacks and strokes.

ELECTROCARDIOGRAM & CARDIOKYMOGRAPHY: It's an EKG and CKG graph that records heart electrical activity. The heart has an electric current running through it. The heart contracts and pumps blood throughout your body. This contraction is started off by an electric current, even though it is a weak one. This current begins in a part of the heart called the sino-atrial node, or the pacemaker, which sets the pace for the heart to beat. From the pacemaker this current follows a well-defined path through the rest of the heart. This movement can be recorded by electrodes, which are plastic plates placed on the chest and limbs to detect current flow inside the heart. The graph recorded is the **EKG and CKG, both painless tests.** These tests detect disturbances in the beating pattern of electrical activity in the heart, called arrhythmia. They also check if any chamber of the heart is abnormally enlarged or if any of the walls have thickened. (See web: *www.Heart.org*)

ECHOCARDIOGRAPHY: This painless ultrasound is used to evaluate structural conditions of the heart like the thickness of the walls; the way the heart walls move during exercise or rest; diagnose valve trouble; inflammation; congenital heart disease and congestive heart failure.

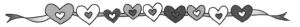

Man's body was created according to the laws of physics and chemistry, which are the Creator's laws. They never vary. His law is written upon every nerve, muscle and faculty which has been entrusted to us.
– Henry W. Vollmer, M.D.

Doctors may now be able to detect "silent" heart disease when CKG test is used with electrocardiograms (EKGs). Recent study revealed EKGs alone missed 39% of heart disease cases. When CKG test was added to EKGs, only 8% of cases went undetected.

182

It uses high-frequency sound waves to produce images of the heart. A small transducer, like a microphone, passes over the chest, sending out impulses that bounce off the heart. The transducer records these echoes, and a computer converts them into a graphic display on the screen.

EndoPAT: Calcium scoring of your coronary arteries: it's an ultrasound measurement taken of the medial thickness of the carotid arteries, which assesses vascular health of the lining of the arteries and small vessels.

Exercise Stress Test: An exercise EKG electrocardiogram that is performed with controlled exercise such as a treadmill. A patient's maximum heart rate is calculated based on their sex and age, then the patient is connected to an EKG machine and exercises until the heart is beating steadily at the calculated rate. This test shows changes in their EKG pattern, especially for those with narrowing of the coronary arteries. If blood pressure drops during the test, this could be another sign of coronary artery disease. The stress test is also used for people who recently recovered from a heart attack, as an initial step in assessing the heart's blood supply. Please express any sensations experienced during the testing (sometimes it's too much too soon). This test can detect coronary artery disease in 75% of cases.

Nuclear Scanning: This safe technique uses radioactive materials known as isotopes, to examine the heart. The isotopes used are harmless substances, and are less radioactive than most x-rays. In nuclear scanning, the patient is given a small dose, either orally or injected. These isotopes flow through the blood system giving off radiation which is photographed by a special camera producing pictures of the heart. These pictures show how well the ventricles are working and where there is scarring, damaged or oxygen-starved areas of the heart.

Stop your life from an out-of-control downward spiral!
Become the Health Captain of your precious life by following
The Bragg Healthy Lifestyle – start today! - Patricia Bragg

There is no thrill quite like doing something you didn't know you could.
– Marjorie Holmes, inspirational author

HOLTER MONITOR: is a portable version of an EKG. It records heart rhythm (pulse) during your daily activities. Worn for 24-72 hours, the heart waves are picked up by electrodes or patches placed on chest. Waves are recorded on tape inside the monitor. This recording is then scanned into a computer for analysis. Holter Monitors are used on patients who experience chest pain, dizziness, palpitations or fainting, which is often caused by narrowing of arteries or heartbeat abnormalities. It may also show evidence of silent ischemia, like an angina attack (page 17) without chest pain. (web: *www.HeartSite.com*)

New Millennium Health Technology Provides Safer, Faster, Better Testing

DIGITAL TECHNOLOGY: can take a routine test like a chest x-ray to a new height of quality and has many advantages. It's an environment saver because there are no film processing chemicals utilized; it is safer for the patient since it uses lower x-ray doses and reduces the need for retakes and more exposure; gives an instant picture and can be stored on a computer and transmitted instantaneously to the doctor's office, the hospital or anywhere required! (See web: *www.MayoClinic.com*)

PET SCANNER: **Positron Emission Tomography** is a unique 32-ring scanner that can detect and measure metabolic activity throughout the body and especially the brain. It pinpoints the source of cancers, neurological and heart diseases; thereby reducing all the expensive, unneeded operations, exploratory surgery and hospital stays! The PET scanner saves time, money and most important, precious lives! (See web: *www.RadiologyInfo.org*)

The more natural food you eat, the more you'll enjoy radiant health and longevity and be able to promote the higher life of love and brotherhood.
– Patricia Bragg, Pioneer Health Crusader

What usually raises your LDL Particle Number is a diet high in processed foods; refined sugars; fast foods; lack of exercise and sleep. – mercola.com

Use your willpower and better judgement to select and eat only foods which are best for you, regardless of any ridicule or gibes of friends. – Dr. Richard T. Field

184

GammaKnife Stereotactic Radiosurgery: (used for surgery) uses a *radionic invisible blade,* not a scalpel; this makes surgery non-invasive, bloodless, and reduces complications, discomfort, and hastens recovery. Excellent for brain tumors and vascular and arteriovenous malformations (AVMs).

Alternate Procedure to Open Heart Surgery

The AngioVac Procedure is a new technological procedure done to remove long blood clots (venous thromboembolism), using a device that suctions out the solid matter of the clot without requiring a blood transfusion! This minimally invasive procedure is considered as a breakthrough and alternative to open-heart surgery.

To do the procedure surgeons first feed a small camera down the throat to monitor the heart. Next, they insert a tube through an artery in the neck and into the heart, with the end pressed against the clot. They thread the other end of the tube through a vein in the groin, and hook the tube up to a heart-bypass machine, which provides suction. When opened, the tip of the *AngioVac* tube captures the blood clot, along with any solid materials. The blood is then filtered and fed back into the body through the vein near the groin, eliminating the need for a blood transfusion.

185

This procedure has been used since 2013 and may be a great option for an older or frail person who could be at high risk for open-heart surgery.

The only thing that is truly yours that no one can take away from you is your attitude. So if you take care of that, everything else in life becomes much easier.

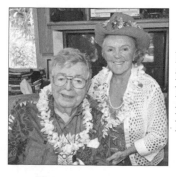

Dr. Earl Bakken with Patricia. He was famous for inventing the first transistor pacemaker. His firm Medtronic, developed it and a resuscitator for fixing ailing hearts that have and are saving thousands of lives!

EECP Therapy Offers Relief for Chest Pain

Enhanced External CounterPulsation Therapy (EECP) is a procedure performed on individuals with chest pain, poor blood flow, angina or heart failure or *cardiomyopathy* in order to diminish their symptoms, improve functional capacity and quality of life. EECP Therapy is a very safe treatment option which generally poses no risk or potential complications to a patient as compared to traditional invasive cardiac procedures.

You may be a candidate for EECP if you have *chronic stable angina*, are not receiving adequate relief from angina by taking nitrates and you do not qualify as a candidate for invasive procedures (bypass surgery, stenting, etc.). Also if you have symptoms of chest pain, shortness of breath and chronic fatigue from walking or physical activity you can be a good candidate for treatment!

During treatment, the patient's legs are wrapped in compressive pneumatic cuffs. The devices squeeze and release – inflating and deflating – to the beat of heart, pushing oxygenated blood toward the heart and into the coronary arteries. The mechanical treatment can encourage and promote growth of new vessels around narrowed and blocked arteries of the heart. These new paths have profound benefits by restoring blood flow of oxygenated blood to the heart. This restoration of nutrient rich blood flow revives tissues in parts of the heart and body that have become "stunned" due to restricted or blocked blood flow. The heart benefits greatly as patients will see an improvement in symptoms of chest pain, shortness of breath, chronic fatigue as well as significant improvement in exercise and energy!

The typical treatment lasts 1-2 hours. Patients undergo 35 hours of EECP therapy, five days a week over 7-weeks. *"The treatment is generally well tolerated and angina symptoms were improved in 75-80% of patients,"* stated American Heart Association.

Many patients who undergo heart surgery suffer significant and long-lasting loss of brain power. It's better to follow Dr. Dean Ornish, and other wise doctors and The Bragg Healthy Lifestyle – who advocate a 100% healthy lifestyle.

Don't let cardiovascular disease affect you! Protect your heart! – please start now!

Chapter 20

Chelation Therapy

What Mainly Causes "Ageing"?

As we discussed earlier in this book, the so-called *ageing process* is not the result of the passage of time, it is primarily the result of inadequate blood circulation, which can and does occur at any calendar age. *The chief villains are an excess of inorganic minerals, calcium, etc. and toxic chemicals (of which undistilled drinking water is a primary source), combined with an excess of cholesterol from a diet rich in saturated animal fats, hydrogenated fats and living an unhealthy lifestyle. All add to the ageing process.*

Arteriosclerosis, or hardening of the arteries, can result from calcium deposits on the arterial walls. With the onset of deadly atherosclerosis, the calcified walls are further thickened by waxy deposits of cholesterol, which then dangerously narrow the blood passageway.

This abnormal calcium acts as a cementing agent and forms plaques with other inorganic minerals, and cholesterol and other waxy fats. This narrowing of the passageway, lessens both the quantity and force of the blood flow. Body cells degenerate from lack of nourishment and slowly drown in their own toxins, causing cells to die!

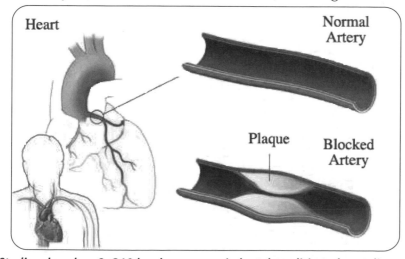

Studies show low CoQ10 levels cause periodontal conditions, heart disease, declining memory and brain function. CoQ10 helped reverse these conditions.
— Dr. Stephen T. Sinatra, author, "CoQ10 Phenomenon," and
"The Sinatra Solution, Metabolic Cardiology"

Chelation – Safe, Effective and Inexpensive Treatment For Coronary Heart Disease

Chelation Therapy is a therapeutic adaptation of a natural biochemical process. The term *chelation* derives from the Greek word *chele* (pronounced keely) meaning a crab-like, pulling claw. Without going into detailed chemistry, chelation in human metabolism is the process by which an enzyme grabs or *binds* an organic mineral or *metal* and transports it to the body part where it can be utilized or removed. Example: Zinc to the pancreas for making insulin; and iron for the hemoglobin (red blood cells); calcium for building bones and its many other body uses. (Remember, this refers to organic minerals – not inorganic, which cannot be used.)

This natural chelation process was not discovered until the 1940s. Its first therapeutic application was during World War II after a synthetic chelating agent was created to act as an antidote for *mustard gas* and other forms of arsenic poisoning. (For 20 years thereafter, chelation [pulling] agents were developed almost exclusively for ridding the body of toxic heavy metals such as lead.)

In the late 1950s chelating agents used as poison antidotes were also effective in removing inorganic calcium deposits from the body's joints, organs and cardiovascular system. Through studies and medical research, a safe, effective chelating agent, known as EDTA was produced for removing these inorganic calcium clogging deposits and cholesterol plaques from the arteries and flushing them out via the kidneys.

EDTA, a natural amino acid chelating agent, does not affect the normal organic calcium utilized by the body, but chelates only pathological inorganic calcium deposits. Chelation has proven for some to be an effective way to reverse hardening of the arteries. It unclogs the arteries by chelating out these atherosclerotic plaques, which then dissolve and break up. The cholesterol and other deposits then become slushy and are easily flushed out. All the residue *goes down the drain* and then the *pipes* of your cardiovascular system become more free flowing.

Chelation Therapy Includes a Healthy Diet

Carlos P. Lamar, M.D. pioneered chelation therapy in the 1960s and developed the basic procedures which included the proper dosage of Endrate (ETDA) – delivered slowly and intravenously, lasting from 3 to 4 hours per treatment.

As an essential part of chelation treatment, Dr. Lamar and his colleagues prescribed an anti-atherogenic diet that naturally chelates. Patients eat more frequent, lighter meals (with more tropical fruits; bananas, kiwis, mangos, papayas and pineapples, rich in the enzyme bromelain that acts like cardiovascular pipe cleaners) and eliminate dairy foods and saturated fats. Emphasis is placed on fresh, organic fruits and vegetables and natural foods.

He also gave them 50 to 100 mg. of vitamin B6 (pyridoxine) to control sodium/potassium blood levels, that help produce red blood cells and hemoglobin and protect against infection, plus additional vitamin and mineral supplements for each patient as needed.

Safe Diagnosis with Non-Invasive Tests

189

All patients are given thorough physicals and tests before the start of chelation therapy, and carefully monitored during the chelation treatments, along with receiving complete instruction for follow-up procedures. An infrared thermographic scan, which is diagnostic equipment, provides a safe, accurate method of locating and determining the degree of arterial blockage. Formerly this was done only by an angiogram test. This scan is a heat-sensitive instrument which records body temperature with direct correlation to blood circulation. This thermogram reveals the location and degree of blockage by a light spectrum with a 10-color range. We endorse the non-invasive tests and infrared thermographic scans listed on pages 181 to 185.

It's good that modern technology is available if you need it, but it's even better to prevent your arteries from getting plugged up in the first place.

Patricia Bragg Books can be your faithful health guides by your side night and day.

We must always change, renew, rejuvenate; otherwise, we harden.
– Johann Wolfgang von Goethe, German poet, playwright, author

Chelation Therapy Promotes Natural Healing

Because it attacks the basic cardiovascular problem of degeneration, chelation therapy helps regenerate the body's natural self-healing and repairing powers. Natural blood circulation then restores normal metabolism and biochemical functions. The whole body *comes alive.*

When the first cases were reported back in 1964 by Dr. Lamar in the national medical publication *Angiology* (Vol. 15, No. 9, Sept. 1964), the most surprising result was the significant decrease in the insulin requirement of diabetics in response to chelation therapy. Two of the early cases were elderly diabetics with extreme mental deterioration and severe cardiovascular complications. After treatment there was a complete remission of symptoms, both physical and mental – plus a marked decrease in their insulin requirement. This *bonus* was attributed to the increased circulation in the pancreas, which promoted insulin production.

190

Since then, chelation therapy has been found to achieve *benefits* for some, such as regeneration and re-hardening of bones weakened by osteoporosis, restoration of mobility to frozen osteoarthritic joints, relief from hypothyroidism, reversal of prostatic calcinosis, recovery of normal functions of the kidney, other glands and organs and improvement in deteriorated retinas. There was improvement in all pathological conditions resulting from impaired circulation.

Chelation (ETDA) treatment has also been effective for some in treating heart disease, and for patients suffering from Multiple Sclerosis and Parkinson's disease. Perhaps the most spectacular results of chelation therapy are evidenced by the restored mental acuity in advanced senility cases.

In a landmark study, Dr. Carlos Lamar stated in the *Journal of American Geriatric Society* (Vol. XIV, No. 3, 1966), *"The physical rehabilitation and enjoyment of living experienced by these patients would be impossible to match through any other available therapeutic procedure."*

A light, happy heart lives longer. – William Shakespeare

A Universal Need for Chelation Therapy

As early as 1968, Dr. Lamar predicted, *"I have little doubt that eventually new ligands (chelating agents) will be created that will be effective by the oral (natural supplements) route.* * *That will be the big step that will bring chelation therapy to the reach of any patient suffering from any form of calcific disease, plaque and cholesterol build-up."*

"The great advance in preventive medicine lies in keeping the arteries open and clean BEFORE the symptoms or attack which make the disorder obvious to everybody," Dr. Evers declared. *"This is where chelation therapy has its greatest future."*

There are hundreds of chelation clinics in America and around the world. The best web source of doctors for chelation therapy is ACAM (the American College for Advancement in Medicine), visit web: *www.acam.org*.

The Benefits of Chelation Therapy

Chelation Therapy helps halt bad effects of ageing and heart disease and initiates the body's healing process, often reversing the damage. Some of the benefits are:

191

- ***Reduces Free Radical Activity in Blood:*** Research shows EDTA can have antioxidant nutrients – vitamins A, C and E, selenium, and amino acid complexes. These not only mop up free radicals but also assist in reinforcing the stability of cell membranes (see pages 25-30).

- ***Blocks Calcium Absorption, Helps Repair Damaged Muscles, Improves the Cell Energy Production:*** EDTA removes the toxic metal ions such as lead, calcium, mercury, cadmium, copper, iron, and aluminum from the blood stream. By removing the extra calcium from the blood stream, there is no more free calcium available to produce plaque. It means that the cells can start to repair themselves. Their production of energy increases. As more and more cells rebuild, our body becomes healthier. They can ward off intruders. The

The heart that loves is always young. – Greek proverb

---

*Health Stores now have oral chelation supplements and Niacin (B3).

result is that we have started a salvage and regeneration activity that repairs previously damaged muscles and the heart and the whole body benefits as a result.

- ***Reduces Blood Stickiness or Clotting:*** EDTA helps to reduce blood platelet formation. This makes the blood less sticky, so the blood can then flow through narrow arteries. It can flow through even partially blocked arteries minimizing the effect of the blockage.

- ***Normalizes Abnormal Cholesterol and HDL Levels:*** Researchers have found that an EDTA infusion, combined with vitamin and mineral supplements, raised the good (HDL) cholesterol and lowered the bad (LDL) cholesterol. If the HDL was low, it was raised; however, if it was already high, its level remained the same. Similarly, the LDL was lowered if it was high. EDTA optimizes the ratio of HDL and LDL.

- ***Mental Health:*** Researchers have noticed that patients who have undergone chelation treatment are less depressed. They were more alert, alive and happier, and had better concentration, memory and more energy.

CHELATION IMPROVES BLOOD FLOW WITHOUT SURGERY:
Atherosclerosis, the narrowing and stiffening of arteries due to accumulation of pathologic calcium and plaque, is the primary cause of diminished circulation and oxygen to our cells. EDTA Chelation Therapy is a cost-effective method for avoiding surgery, that enhances health of the arteries, removing pathologic calcium, improving elasticity, thus improving circulation and health.

Now, stop and think! Our Creator presented you with the world's most miraculous machine – your own body! This incredible factory has its own non-stop motor (heart), its own fueling system (digestive system), its own filtration system (kidneys), its own thinking computer (brain and nervous system), its own temperature controls (sweat glands), etc. Indeed, this miraculous creation even has the power to reproduce itself!

Health is the most natural thing in the world. It is natural to be healthy because we are a part of Mother Nature – we are nature. Nature is trying hard to keep us well, because she needs us in her business.
– Elbert G. Hubbard, American writer, artist and philosopher, 1856-1915

A Harvard Study shows the strong importance of mind/body connections in your health. Improving your mind with meditation, prayer, relaxation, walking, yoga, healthy diet, some fasting and positive thinking brought amazing improvements.

Chapter 21

The Healthful Art of Longevity

The best recipe for a long life is to keep living The Bragg Healthy Lifestyle. There is no substitute for this!

Consider each day a little life in itself – make it as perfect and well-rounded as you can! Try to have a stronger heart and better health on your next birthday than you have today! By living supremely in each moment you are living superbly for a long, healthy, happy, fulfilled future!

You must always be self-aware of your life! The moment you relax your guard the enemy is ready to rush in and smite you in your heart. True, with luck, you may live long without trying, but you will live longer and better if you exert effort! Healthy living for longevity is an art. Those who deliberately set out to prolong their days have a healthy chance of doing just that!

Forgetfulness of self may make the time go like magic, but it does not help build a strong heart and keep you youthful. Inattention to yourself and the carelessness that results is extremely dangerous! As you live longer you should grow less objective and more subjective. The more self-centered you are, the better you will conserve your precious health resources! Longevity often belongs not to those who forget themselves for others, but to those who are most health conscious of themselves and their physical, mental, spiritual and emotional well-being!

193

This may seem to give the long-lived a positive, strong, and at times selfish character. Not at all! Without healthy nourishment we cannot aspire to fulfill our dreams. To seek to prolong one's life is to extend one's term of usefulness and service! We aren't advocating you prolong your life at the expense of others! Rather, we suggest that you live a long, healthy life so that you may be more useful to your family and others, as well as to yourself!

It's important that people know what you stand for. It's equally important that they know what you won't stand for! – Mary Waldrip

---

A man is as old as his arteries – his river of life. – Thomas Sydenham, English Physician (1624-1689) also known as "English Hippocrates"

Secret of Longevity – Obey Mother Nature

The secret of longevity is to understand that *the enemy is not your chronological age. Premature ageing is preventable!* You must put up a strong defense against ageing. You might find a few octogenarians who say they owe their long life to smoking, alcohol and avoiding exercise. You can tell them confidently that they could extend their lifespan by a good 20 years by living a healthy lifestyle.

Scientific longevity is based on a knowledge of the body and the laws of health. Above all, it means reliance on Mother Nature. She abhors ill health, which is another name for toxic poisoning and clogged pipes. She is always striving to purify and to vitalize. She wants to help you if you will only let her. Medicine, drugs and doctors will do you no good if Mother Nature is not backing them up!

Heart Disease is Your Greatest Threat

Remember that you must always defend yourself against coronary thrombosis (heart attack), stroke, hypertension (high blood pressure), arteriosclerosis (hardening of arteries), atherosclerosis (blockage and clogging of the arteries by cholesterol and other debris), angina pectoris, varicose veins and other cardiovascular (heart and blood vessel) diseases. *Diseases of the heart and circulatory system are the #1 Killer in the United States*! And never forget that you must also guard against stiffening joints, fibrous tissues, deafness, blindness and many other enemies of health and life.

All this means that there must be a little slowing of activity. We believe the advice *grow old gracefully* is wrong! Mother Nature and God will eventually decree the end – but until then it's far better to live life as youthfully as possible! You are *as old as you feel – so feel young!* When you abide by Mother Nature's Laws, you feel younger! By trusting in and obeying Her laws, understanding your miracle physical machine and how to care for it, you can live a longer, more youthful, healthy, happy life.

194

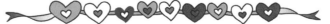

*Smiles increase your face value! A genuine smile is love
you give to yourself and others.*

#1 Cause of Death – Coronary Disease

Deposits in the arteries retard the circulation of blood. The speed and efficiency of the bloodstream has a great effect upon the prolongation of life. It is the bloodstream which provides the entire body with required nourishment and oxygen before it removes harmful substances for elimination. Slowing of blood circulation, loss of elasticity of blood vessels and disturbances of the machinery which regulate distribution of blood are among the most important causes of the shortening of life, vigor and health.

In our opinion, there is no physiological principle limiting health or human lifespan. We believe that radiant health and youthfulness is within reach, but it must be earned. This is your life! It is your sacred duty to yourself to learn now and how to keep your body healthy and fit for a long lifetime!

The #1 cause of widows and widowers in the United States is coronary (heart) disease. Remember our discourse of cholesterol, and the fact that high cholesterol levels are invitations to heart attacks? Statistics show that cholesterol levels in American men and women increase rapidly between ages 30 and 65. Be on guard!

195

Women before the age of 50 used to be much better protected against degenerative artery disease than men. Today women have achieved an unfortunate equality by developing heart attacks and strokes with more frequency than men. The scientific theory that female sex hormones play an important part in providing protection against the harmful menace of atherosclerosis is apparently true – but not powerful enough to offset the deadly effects of an unhealthy lifestyle! (See risks and symptoms for women pages 55-58). As soon as menopause starts in women, the protection of these sex hormones ceases, and they become just as susceptible as men to heart attacks and strokes. It's important, women of all ages should not neglect their heart health.

Roses are God's autograph of beauty, fragrance and love.
– Paul C. Bragg, N.D., Ph.D.

Dr. Paul Dudley White of Boston – Famous Heart Specialist's Wise Words

Dr. White, a founder and former president of the American Heart Association, world famous pioneer heart specialist and our friend, gave this advice on taking care of the heart. We want to call attention especially to the following points made by Dr. White in an article written for the American Heart Association. He begins with his startling facts that *middle age begins at 20,* and the *dangerous years are ages 20 to 40!*

When asked, when does middle age begin?, Dr. White responded *"At age 20, and lasts until 80. And the dangerous years of this span are the first 20 years, not the last. These are the years when an overfed and under-exercised public is sowing the seeds of a coronary harvest! I conceive the ages of man as five. Birth to 20th year; then a three stage middle age of 20 to 40, 40 to 60, 60 to 80; and finally old age – 80 to 100. Latter constitutes a steadily expanding horizon which I see no eventual limit. Our life expectancy should keep rising indefinitely as research keeps making progress against disease."*

Unlimited Life Expectancy is Possible!

Dr. White additionally stated, *"The public can play an important role in this effort to push life-span farther and farther. Physical-fitness and nutritional programs for men and women between ages of 24 and 40 would guard against creeping degeneration and would instill lifelong good health habits!"*

"A man marries sometime in his 20s; his wife cooks too much and too well – and between her cooking, the family car, and the television, man has gained maybe 20-40 pounds by the time he's 45. These are the years in which atherosclerosis (cholesterol blocking and clogging the arteries) and rusting of the arteries occur. This can ultimately reach the brain as a stroke, or heart as a coronary thrombosis (massive blood clot). It may also affect kidneys. This is why an apparently healthy man drops dead at 45 or 50. His death is not sudden at all; an unhealthy lifestyle has silently been building up for years!"

"The automobile and the television, I might add, should be the servants of the American public, not its masters. Despite the nation's generally unhealthy way of life, two factors work in favor of the American person," Dr. White concludes. *"It is never too late – at any age – to begin controlling obesity and resuming a program of sensible exercise and a healthy diet. One excellent form, available to all, is walking! This should be brisk, and for a normally healthy person five miles weekly is not enough. Neither is one weekly 18-hole golf game."*

There you have it – from Dr. Dudley White, known as Dean of American Cardiology. Exercise and diet can be regular and enjoyable parts of a healthy lifestyle as you will discover by following this Bragg Heart Fitness Program we are outlining for you.

Dr. Carrel's Successful Eternal Life Study

Dr. Alexis Carrel, eminent biologist and Nobel Laureate, of the Rockefeller Institute of Medical Research *proved* to the world that *living flesh can be deathless!* In 1912, this Nobel Scientist took a sliver of a heart muscle from a chicken embryo and provided it with 2 essentials of life – simple protein food and correct drainage for the tissues. His simple laboratory experiment kept this tiny piece of embryo heart flesh tissues alive for 35 years.

197

This 35 year study proved that the heart tissue could have continued indefinitely! In 1912, Dr. Carrell received the Nobel Prize for this cell biology work. At the end of the experiment in 1947, this heart tissue had lived many average chicken lifetimes – the equivalent of hundreds of years of human life! It was called the *tissue of eternal youth.*

This amazing bit of embryo heart flesh doubled its size every 48 hours! Slices had to be cut away and discarded daily because its continued growth would have made it impossible to feed and cleanse the living heart cells. At the Rockefeller Institute, any scientist could observe eternal life before their very eyes! We can learn an important lesson from Dr. Carrel's revealing scientific demonstration with tissues from a chicken heart. Namely, that if the body is correctly fed and its poisons and wastes are properly eliminated, life can continue indefinitely! (*www.NobelPrize.org*)

Control Your Biological "Clock Of Life"

You can only get sound health from your healthy circulating blood being nourished by correct food, liquids and air. These substances must be actively distributed throughout your body by the heart and blood vessels.

It is our contention that any person – regardless of age or physical condition – can rebuild themselves and have a stronger heart with cleaner *pipes*. My father demonstrated this with his own body. His abundant health, strength, endurance and stamina were the best proof of the success. He rebuilt his body from a hopeless, physical wreck into a sound, healthy and efficient cardiac human miracle machine with vigorous cardiovascular circulation.

Age is not a matter of how many years you have lived! It resolves itself into how clean your arteries are and the health condition of your blood. You can control your own biological *clock of life* . . . and there is no reason why you cannot strive for and fulfill the Biblical prophecy:

Man's days shall be 120 years. – Genesis 6:3

198

"Old Age" is Not Necessary

Do not be discouraged by your physical condition! *Remember that the body is self-repairing, self-healing and self-maintaining. Where there's life, there's hope!* Working with Mother Nature, you can start to rebuild a healthy bloodstream, and this will help you build a fit heart. To live long you must have a strong heart and clean blood vessels that are flexible, unclogged and elastic. *This Bragg Healthy Heart Fitness Program is your Blueprint to a New You with vital, fresh Super Health!*

Why grow old? *Old age* is not necessary – at least not as necessary as you may think. Instead of submissively growing old – *revolt! Grow young* – you can defy time! At 60 you can be bright-eyed as a bird and radiate the joy of living. At 70 you can be supple, youthful and full of sunny cheer. At 80 you can wear age like a jewel.

In a Harvard Alumni Study, walking 2 miles a day, 7 days a week, produced the highest protection to stay healthy and not have a heart attack!

Turn Back the Clock! Be Healthy and Youthful, follow The Bragg Healthy Lifestyle!

Paul C. Bragg & Mentor – Bernarr Macfadden

My dad worked closely with Bernarr Macfadden and together they changed the entire health culture in America. While Dad was the father of the Health Movement and the originator of health food stores, Macfadden was known as the father of physical culture in America. He founded the *"Physical Culture Magazine,"* the first of its kind in the country. My father served as the editor of the magazine, which brought the basic principles of healthful living to popular attention in America. They were credited with "getting women out of bloomers into shorts, and men into bathing trunks." Macfadden started "Penny Kitchen Restaurants" during the big Depression Era, when they fed millions of hungry people for a penny each. Bragg helped Macfadden with his Miami Health Spa Hotel: The Macfadden – Deauville Hotel.

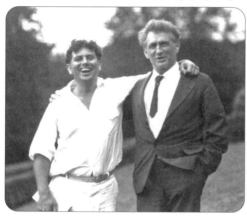

Paul Bragg & Mentor – Bernarr Macfadden

My dad was associated for many years with Macfadden, who spent thousands of dollars to find the oldest living humans on earth. Dad was his main researcher on this project. This took him to many very interesting, remote parts of the world, interviewing men and women from 103 to 120 years of age! Dad found this work fascinating, because he loved promoting health and longevity, and not just the life of the average person which ends at about 77, but an active life that would last 120 to 150 years (Genesis 6:3). The Bragg research proved it can be done! Now Scientists worldwide are agreeing.

Researchers have discovered the more healthy habits an individual practices, the longer they live and the healthier they are! – Elizabeth Vierck, "Health Smart"

Slow down and enjoy life. It's not only the scenery you miss by going too fast, you also miss the sense of where you're going and why! – Eddie Cantor, Hollywood

---

What you eat and drink or whatever you do
– do it all to the glory of God and your human temple – your body.
– 1 Corinthians 10:31 and 3 John 2 are Patricia Bragg's mottos

---

You are what you eat, drink, breathe, think, say and do. – Patricia Bragg

Life's Quantity and Quality Depends Upon the Food We Eat and Our Activity

We've learned a great deal about keeping the heart fit by means of a simple natural food diet and vigorous exercise.

We know that when the mass of civilized, humankind adopts a simple natural diet with exercise and keeping active, then there will be more people who will reach remarkable ages. Every intelligent person will agree that life's length and quality depends largely upon the food we eat. How carefully we select our foods will logically depend on how sound our heart, brain, nerves, body cells, tissues and vital organs will be tomorrow, next month, next year and 10 years from now! *The chemistry of the food a person eats becomes the chemistry of their body.*

Old Age is Not Inevitable – Scientists Say Man Should Live to 140 to 185

It seems to us that what we call *old age* is the result of sluggish cell action in the body. The cells are being renewed all the time by the moisture in the lymph circulation, just as a tree is renewed all the time by the circulation of its sap. But if the cell is clogged in any way by toxic deposits which it cannot be completely rid of – chiefly because of poor blood circulation – it cannot then make full use of the building material brought by the lymphatic system or the new health nourishment and oxygen delivered by the bloodstream.

Biologists tell us that man grows an entirely new body every 11 months. That being the case, why does mankind age? Scientists answer this by saying that the body fails to shed all of the old cells. As we stated earlier, deposits in the cell prevent its full use of the new material. So instead of living 7 times the period it takes man to mature, as most animals do, man's life is unnaturally shortened by his unhealthy lifestyle. Sad facts!

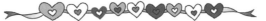

Scientists may be able to make substantial gains in extending not only the length of human life, but the quality of life as we age, that won't be limited to breakthroughs in the laboratory. To a significant extent, longevity depends on how we live our lives!

Conrad Hilton Thanks Bragg for His Long Life!

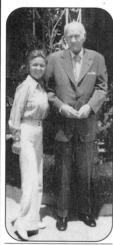

Patricia with Conrad Hilton

When the world's most famous hotel magnate, Conrad Hilton, was 80 years old and lying on his deathbed, we gave him a new lease on life by introducing him to The Bragg Healthy Lifestyle. He followed our instructions and discovered a whole new healthy, vibrant lifestyle! He was soon healthy, happy and fit, enjoying life! He even remarried at 88 years young! He remained active in business (half days at his office) into his 90's!! Mr. Hilton, at 88, was quoted in a *People Magazine* interview as saying, *"I wouldn't be alive today if it wasn't for the Braggs and their Bragg Healthy Lifestyle!"* Here's a photo of the grateful hotel founder with his healthy lifestyle teacher, Patricia Bragg.

Unhealthy Lifestyle Living is Slow Suicide

Just because you are *feeling fine* does not mean you can afford the risk of continuing to choke your bloodstream with the high cholesterol diet typical of most people in our *modern* civilization. Bacon and eggs, meat, potatoes, pies and cakes, bread with butter or margarine, milk and ice cream, all the rich foods that most men and women crave are slow poisons to your heart and circulatory system! Remember that these poisons work silently and insidiously. Their effect may not become evident until you suddenly have a heart attack. Always remember the wise words of famous Dr. Paul D. White:

"Death from a heart attack is not sudden,
it had been building up for years by
your lifestyle and eating habits!"

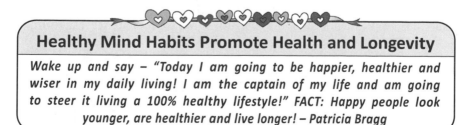

Healthy Mind Habits Promote Health and Longevity

Wake up and say – "Today I am going to be happier, healthier and wiser in my daily living! I am the captain of my life and am going to steer it living a 100% healthy lifestyle!" FACT: Happy people look younger, are healthier and live longer! – Patricia Bragg

Your Family's Life is in Your Hands

We would like to suggest to everyone that you re-read Dr. White's warning and you take it seriously. If you want to keep your family healthy, inspire them to exercise every day as you watch what you feed them and yourself!

Remember that young people can also die of heart disease! Teach your children how to eat correctly! Give your family more fresh salads, more lightly steamed vegetables, more fresh fruit desserts. Eliminate dairy products. Enjoy healthier soy, rice and nut milks. Serve delicious herbal teas such as mint, chamomile, lemon balm and banish the salt shaker from your table! Your reward will be a radiantly happy, healthy family.

Enjoy Lighter, Smaller Vegetarian Dinners

It seems to be an American custom for people to eat their biggest meal in the evening. From a standpoint of heart attacks, this is the worst time to eat a big meal . . . especially a meal with a preponderance of fat. It has been definitively established by researchers that the blood is more likely to clot 2 to 8 hours following a meal with a high fat intake. It would therefore seem logical to avoid heavy meals – particularly in the evening – to minimize the chances of intravascular clotting. The occurrence of a heart attack after eating a heavy meal has been recognized by doctors for years. Just think how often you read or hear about a man in his prime dying of a heart attack during his sleep at night or in the morning.

Eat Plenty of Raw Cabbage – A Miracle Cleanser and Healer

Cabbage (raw) has amazing properties. It stimulates the immune system, kills bacteria and viruses, heals ulcers, and according to Dr. James Balch in "Prescription for Cooking and Dietary Wellness", your chances of contracting colon cancer can be reduced by 60% by eating cabbage weekly. Dr. Saxon-Graham states that those who never consume cabbage were three times more likely to develop colon cancer. A Japanese study shows that people who ate cabbage had the lowest fatality rate from any cancer. Therapeutic benefits have also been attributed to cabbage in relation to scurvy, gout, rheumatism (arthritis), eye diseases, asthma, pyorrhea and gangrene. See Patricia's Raw Organic Vegetable Health Salad recipe page 151. We love cabbage and also we make a variety of sandwiches wrapped in cabbage leaves instead of bread.

Retired people, of course, can regulate their meal-times easily. Business people can dine at an earlier hour in the evening and can certainly regulate their diet to promote their health and prolong their lives!

A light healthy vegetarian meal is ideal for evenings.

It can begin with a raw combination salad with lemon and olive oil dressing. Follow it with 2 lightly cooked vegetables such as green beans, zucchini, peas, corn on the cob, kale, okra, vegetable chop suey, etc. Several nights a week add a baked potato – but do not drench this potato in fat! Season it with fresh garlic and herbs or sea kelp and drizzle with organic olive oil instead of butter.

Now we are not telling you that the price you must pay to avoid a heart attack and live a longer life is to give up good flavor. Not at all!

You Can Teach Old Dogs New Tricks

They say you *can't teach an old dog new tricks.* We feel wise, mature humans have the intelligence to protect themselves from heart attacks by learning new tricks of eating! Start now improving your daily lifestyle habits! 203

To avoid heart attacks you must learn to substitute organic extra virgin olive oil instead of butter, margarine and other clogging, saturated and hydrogenated fats. If you are a milk drinker, learn to substitute rice or almond milks and drink these instead of cow's milk. Learn to use fresh herbs and spices, sea kelp, garlic, onions, and coconut aminos to add delicious flavors and aromas instead of salting your foods. Also, remember that saturated fats, hormones and antibiotics in meats, and dairy products are your enemies! Learn to eat them sparingly or not at all. *Keep meals as healthy, natural and simple as possible!*

Most people shake their heads in doubt when they are told they must give up using salt. It does take a little time to make the change from salt, but the cravings will disappear, and you will find that your 260 taste buds will soon reject salted foods.

It's magnificent to live long if one keeps
healthy, alert, youthful and active.
– Harry Emerson Fosdick, American Pastor (1878 – 1969)

Feel Youthful Regardless of Your Years

Life is the survival of the fittest and no one – yes, no one – is going to be able to protect your heart except you! It's your duty and responsibility to yourself to live a healthy lifestyle so that your heart can remain strong and healthy throughout your entire natural lifespan.

We must live by knowledge and wisdom – not by old wives' tales and myths. That is why this book was written: to provide the scientific facts about your heart and outline a *Heart Fitness Program* that helps you take care of your marvelous, life-giving machine.

This book's message is simple. It tells what a heart attack is, what causes it and what you can do today to prevent it. We offer no magic formula or cure for heart trouble. In this Heart Fitness Program we have simply brought together well-documented evidence from the great scientific and medical researchers, statisticians and dietitians of the world. The medical world is relying upon heart transplants, surgeries and drugs. We are not. Instead, we are interested in disease prevention by keeping the heart healthy and fit! Let's stop heart troubles before they start! Why wait for the heart to deteriorate before we do something about it? We must live healthy today, so that we don't have a heart attack tomorrow! What we sow in one period of our lives, we reap in another. Let's sow seeds of good health so that we will automatically have a powerful, fit heart.

You can definitely capture and retain the joyous feeling of youthfulness no matter what your calendar years may be! By living The Bragg Healthy Lifestyle outlined in this Heart Fitness Program, you can again regain the joy of youthfulness and boundless energy.

204

Happiness is not being pained in body or troubled in mind.
– Thomas Jefferson, 3rd U.S. President, 1801-1809

I've seen sickness and asthma disappear completely in response to major shifts in diet and lifestyles, as in eliminating sugar, milk, meat and switching to healthier, vegetarian diet.
– Dr. Andrew Weil

Don't let people drag you down to their low level of thinking. *You are as young as your arteries!* Decide that you are going to live a healthful life to help keep your arteries and heart years younger. Keep your *thinking* youthful and you will feel young again! Age is not birthdays – it's a matter of how well you live, feel and enjoy each day of your life!

You Can "Grow Younger" – It's Up to You

You stand at life's crossroads. Will you take the path of least resistance that often leads to a premature end, or will you climb to the clear heights of a healthful, youthful, radiant life? If you are going to strive for healthy longevity, begin today! Begin right now – don't procrastinate! Regard this Heart Fitness System also as a Program of Inspiration. It's intended to induce you to take stock of your life, get a fresh grip, and hoist yourself onto a higher plane so you can enjoy Health, Happiness and Longevity!

Why not *grow younger?* If you desire this, you will have the power, and by the Great Goddess of Good Health – Hygeia – you will succeed! Our Healthy Heart Fitness Program shows you how to create a powerful heart, a healthy balanced bloodstream and a strong circulatory system. We can't do it for you – You must do it for yourself!

We offer no *specifics* and no *cures*, for only Mother Nature has the power to heal a diseased heart! When you give your bloodstream the proper building materials, you can build a healthier and more fit body to help empower your body to help heal you!

CARDIOVASCULAR DISEASE IS NOT THE INEVITABLE RESULT OF AGEING.
Healthy preventive measures can be taken to avoid heart disease.
– James F. Balch, M.D., co-author "Prescription for Nutritional Healing"

Age does not depend upon years, but upon lifestyle and health!

Our habits, good or bad, are something we should and can control!
– Dr. Edward J. Stieglitz, wrote articles for "Journal of American Medical Association"

Remember – Prevention is always preferable to the cure!

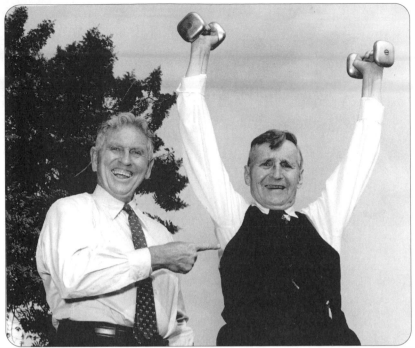

Paul C. Bragg and His Friend Roy White who lived to 106.
My father's good friend, Roy White of Long Beach, California, had a tireless, painless and ageless body. He knew the Laws of Mother Nature and he lived by them. He didn't fear old age. We both could name many more friends who are in their 80s, 90s and even over 100, who are biologically youthful!

Remember that throughout this Bragg Heart Fitness Program we have stressed how important it is to keep physically active. Our claims are backed up by this 106 year old youngster! Don't let your circulation slow down!

To over-rest is to rust and rust can lead to destruction.

Roy believed his daily brisk walks help him physically, mentally, emotionally and spiritually! He believed you can walk off your tensions and worries. Roy said, *I've always been free from tensions – that's the foundation of my Philosophy of Life. Fear and hatred are the two worst things in the world. You can multiply your troubles by thinking they're worse than they are – no matter how mean anyone has been to me, I've never hated them. Let them do the hating, not me!*

To be seventy years young is sometimes far more cheerful and hopeful than to be forty years old. – Oliver Wendell Holmes

Forgiving & Forgetting Keeps You Youthful

Tensions, anger, greed and excessive emotionalism can damage your heart! Roy was an example of the great philosophy of forgiving and forgetting! He says most young children think that way and he always wanted to be kind and think youthful! When you have a strong sense of well-being and optimism, your entire attitude toward life is fresher and more youthful! Your whole philosophy can change to a younger and more optimistic one, replacing the stagnating defeatist attitude many people have. When you feel youthful, you act youthful and then all your actions and thinking are more youthful!

It's Never Too Late to Think Youthfully

This whole Heart Fitness Program is designed to make you forget birthdays and live a more youthful, carefree life. Living by this philosophy of life prevents many physical and mental miseries that are likely to afflict older people. In this way you can maintain health, strength, vigor and happiness as the years roll by. It has been said that *There is really no cure for old age – only those who die young escape it*. But our Heart Fitness Program can really help you feel and look younger and enjoy living longer.

Self improvements have been shown to be effective to help you accept yourself for what you are and feel positive for what you see in yourself and your future goals! Goals practiced daily for about 15 minutes are more productive than spending all your waking hours fighting to lose weight, or other negatives you find in yourself. During self hypnosis (self-guidance) tell yourself to let go all the bad feelings about yourself, breathe deeply, then relax. Concentrate on feeling comfortable about each area of your body and tell yourself to treat yourself more lovingly. When you can forgive yourself, you'll be able to forgive others easier and feel better about yourself and everyone around you! This helps you become motivated into loving action to improve your entire lifestyle on all levels!

It is sad that many people go through life committing partial slow suicide destroying their health, youth, beauty, talents, energies and creative qualities. Indeed, to learn how to be good to oneself is often more difficult than to learn how to be good to others.
– Paul C. Bragg, N.D., Ph.D.

We No Longer Celebrate Birthdays

That is absolutely right. No more birthdays for us! We no longer want to measure our lives by calendar years – only by healthy, biological years! Don't think the years are making you old – it's the way you live that preserves or damages your heart and arteries! You must earn your youthful arteries! You must work hard to preserve the vitality and fitness of your heart and your body! It's wonderful when you buildup a fit heart and body, for then you find more time and energy for so many more activities than you did when you were stumbling around tired and only half-alive. When you have a heart that is beating joyfully, the world looks like the Garden of Eden! You become a carefree person with a song in your heart, a sparkle in your eye and a spring in your step. Life can be beautiful – for when you're healthy, you're happy! After all, is that not the greatest goal in life – *sweet, contented happiness and inner peace!*

208

Health, Happiness and Longevity – It's All Up to You!

The results back up our teachings. You, and only you, can take proper care of your heart and body so that you may enjoy the *prime of your life* indefinitely! Most people reach their *prime* between 25 and 35, and then experience a decline. People who follow this Bragg Heart Fitness Program can attain the prime of life at any age and maintain and enjoy it for life! Now, plan and follow this Program!

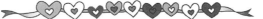

Each birthday is the beginning of your own personal fresh new year! Your first birthday was a beginning, and each birthday is a chance to begin again, to start over, to take a new grip on life. – Paul C. Bragg, N.D., Ph.D., Life Extension Specialist

Positive affirmations create miracles. – Beatrex Quntanna

Nothing transforms a person as much as changing from a negative attitude to a healthy positive attitude!

Now learn what and how a temperate diet will bring great benefits along with it. In the first place, you will enjoy good health. – Horace, 65 B.C.

Man's days shall be to 120 years. – Genesis 6:3

Chapter 22

Herbs & Food Supplements Are Mother Nature's Great Healers

This book gives you a lively lifestyle program for a healthy, rewarding life. When you follow The Bragg Healthy Lifestyle you can build a strong, healthy heart. This will take you down the path to increased well-being confidence, creativity and vitality! Please remember always strive to live a more healthy, happy, positive life!

In building a healthier and stronger heart don't forget the miraculous healing gifts available from Mother Nature's kingdom. For thousands of years people around the world have used herbs and plants as medicines, tonics and remedies. Many of them are renowned for increasing heart health. Today, scientific research supports the traditional use of many of these medicinal plants. Herbs such as garlic, ginkgo, hawthorn, bilberry, gotu kola and rosemary have been traditionally used and scientifically researched for the treatment of heart and circulatory conditions. Following are brief descriptions of some of the most effective herbs, and we encourage you to make use of these miracles of the plant world for your heart's health and fitness. Remember to consult your health care professional before substituting herbs in a previously existing condition. The key to a healthy heart is prevention and The Bragg Healthy Heart Program.

Garlic – This Herb Helps Lower Cholesterol

Garlic is one of nature's great miracles! No other medicinal plant is more effective in the treatment and prevention of atherosclerosis! No wonder there has been increased research involving garlic and cardiovascular health. Research shows eating garlic regularly decreases serum cholesterol and dangerous triglyceride levels! People who eat garlic regularly have healthier arteries and blood than those who don't. This is why people in France, Greece, and Italy (who traditionally eat lots of garlic) have a lower incidence of heart attacks and disease than people in the United States.

Garlic – Your Body's Health Friend

Garlic's health role is protecting your heart. The cloves contain many natural anticoagulants that help thin the blood and help protect against platelet stickiness – thus lowering the risk of clotting and even a stroke! Plus, garlic has potent immune-enhancing properties and may eradicate many types of bacteria and fungi, including salmonella and candida; as well as inhibit gastrointestinal ulcers. (We love garlic with foods.)

In 1993 an extensive revealing study on garlic *(called poor man's penicillin)* in the *Annals of Internal Medicine* found small amounts of fresh garlic eaten daily can significantly lower cholesterol levels in people with high cholesterol levels. Other exciting studies show that garlic helps decrease the blood's bad LDL-cholesterol levels while increasing levels of good HDL-cholesterol! It's also a general blood tonic. Please make fresh garlic part of your daily routine – a clove a day for prevention, 2-3 cloves to lower your cholesterol.

210

Remove garlic's outer papery skin. Let sit 10 minutes after chopping, to let beneficial enzymes develop. Varieties of garlic include: shallots, elephant garlic, Spanish or red garlic, garlic spears – all have great health benefits!

The Healing Powers of Onions

Ancient Egyptians and Romans prized the extraordinary healing powers of onions. Research supports these claims. According to studies, consuming one medium onion a day helps lower your cholesterol by 15%. The onion is rich in sulfur – which helps lower levels of blood fats and keeps plaque from adhering to artery walls. Sulfur is also a powerful detox element, releasing toxins from the liver. Foods naturally high in sulfur also help the body to detox from heavy metals like lead, arsenic and cadmium.

The onion is the richest dietary source of quercetin, a powerful antioxidant flavonoid that has been shown to thin the blood, lower cholesterol, ward off blood clots, fight asthma, chronic bronchitis, hay fever, diabetes, atherosclerosis and infections and is even linked to inhibiting certain cancer types.

Onions come in many varieties: yellow, red (our favorite), white, leeks, chives and scallions – all beneficial to your health! Sweet onions – Vidalia, Maui or Walla Walla have lower sulfur content than other more pungent varieties. To minimize tears, chill onions for half an hour before peeling and chopping. It's best to eat them raw for their full health benefit in salads, dips, spreads, soups and sandwiches. When cooking onions, lightly sauté them, for over-cooking can destroy important enzymes.

Ginkgo – Promotes Blood Flow

Over the last 40 years, Ginkgo has been one of the most scientifically researched medicinal herbs in the world today. Scientists know that *Gingko Biloba* (leaf) *Extracts* (GBE) dilate arteries, capillaries and veins, which increases blood flow. Therefore GBE reduces blood clotting and clogging of the arteries. GBE's strong cardiovascular benefits are localized in the brain. Increasing evidence supports the GBE effectiveness in treating ailments associated with too little blood flow to the brain (such as short-term memory loss, senility, short attention span and depression). In addition, GBE inhibit platelet aggregation, reduce blood clotting and work through antioxidants to protect our vascular walls from free-radical damage (see pages 25-27).

211

Ginkgo Biloba has also been shown to help alleviate the symptoms of other ailments. By improving circulation, the herb can ease dizziness, migraine headaches and the perpetual ringing in the ears that doctors call tinnitus. Some people who take Ginkgo also experience an improvement in their breathing, which reduces the hardening of the arteries that arteriosclerosis causes. Look for Ginkgo Biloba supplements in health stores.

A wise man should consider that health is the greatest of human blessings, and learn how by his own thought to derive benefit from his illnesses. Hippocrates, Father of Medicine, 400 B.C.

Ageing causes a general loss of blood vessel elasticity. This "hardening" effect can cause high blood pressure and increase the likelihood of an occlusion in a blood vessel. Ginkgo provides a "relaxant" effect on blood vessels, thereby increasing their youthful elasticity. – Life Extension Magazine

Hawthorn – Multiple Cardiovascular Benefits

The Hawthorn Berry is used for the treatment of hypertensions, angina, cardiac arrhythmias and congestive heart failure. Scientific studies show hawthorn's ability to dilate blood vessels (especially coronary vessels associated with angina). These effects can be traced to the pigment found in hawthorn flowers, leaves and berries. These phytonutrients include bioflavonoids that have strong antioxidant properties and assist our body in ridding itself of free radicals. They also help our body distribute and effectively use vitamin C and strengthen capillaries. These stronger capillaries and dilated blood vessels allow our heart to better circulate blood, thus delivering oxygen to every system of our body and providing our heart with the nutrients it needs. Hawthorn improves heart cell metabolism and enhances the flow of electrolytes across the cardiac cells. This prevents or corrects heart rhythm abnormalities and strongly encourages a healthy cardiac rhythm. When getting hawthorn, be sure to get the whole plant – leaves, flowers, and berry. The berries contain more proanthocyanidins while the flowers and leaves contain more vitexin. The most effective way to consume hawthorn if you are unable to get it fresh is in a dried and ground form.

Put fresh or dried hawthorn in smoothies, juices, and teas and enjoy daily. It has great antioxidant and cardiovascular boosting effects and is great to use before or after exercise. This improves exercise recovery by improving oxygen flow and neutralizes scavenging free radicals from damaged tissues.

HAWTHORN BERRY: Laboratory studies show that this herb has antioxidant properties that help protect against the formation of plaques, which leads atherosclerosis. Plaque buildup in the vessels that supply the heart with oxygen-rich blood may cause chest pain (angina) and heart attacks while plaque buildup in the arteries that supply blood to the brain may result in stroke.
– HerbWisdom.com/herb-hawthorn-berry.html

Hawthorn Berry helps prevent free radical-induced oxidation of good LDL cholesterol, a step that must occur before LDL can form plaque in the arteries. It was also shown to protect vitamin E from damage and synergistically boost vitamin E status by 18%-20%.

Cayenne – Boosts Circulation & Energizes Heart

People worldwide use a variety of hot peppers in their cooking. Peppers are also firmly rooted in traditions of folk medicine. When we talk of cayenne pepper, we are referring to red hot peppers of the genus, *capsicum annuum* – which includes cayenne, the famous Tabasco pepper, Mexican chili peppers, pimiento, the Louisiana long pepper and others. All contain pungent *capsaicin,* that gives hot pepper its kick and important healthy active ingredients for your circulation and your heart.

Prior to the Civil War the red pepper had gained a reputation in the U.S. as a heat rub when applied to the skin. Since then people have found it promotes health and healing in many ways! Example: cayenne has become popular as a digestive aid and pain reliever salve for sprains, backaches, etc. Also try cayenne and DMSO lotions (pat lightly – don't rub).

Cayenne is a powerful heart and health healer, so make use of it's potential! Studies confirm cayenne's effect as a general blood tonic, linking it to a reduction of blood clotting. These studies show capsaicin (cayenne) has beneficial effects on the cardiovascular system, helps lower cholesterol levels and helps prevent heart disease, see pages 19 and 240. For healthy heart benefits add cayenne flakes to food regularly to season: soups, potatoes, vegetables, salads, beans, rice, etc. instead of salt! *We take one cayenne 40,000 HU capsule daily with meals.* Try this warm drink: stir $1/2$ lemon, tiny pinch cayenne flakes (and honey if desired) in a cup of hot water.

A Japanese study has linked cayenne (capsaicin) pepper intake with improved oxygen levels in the blood. This helps keep your heart and cardiovascular system open and your brain and memory more alert.

HERBS & SUPPLEMENTS FOR HEALTHY HEART: Cayenne powder and tincture, Hawthorn Berry tinctures, Gotu Kola extracts, Evening Primrose Oil, Motherwort, Magnesium, Red Sage, Cinnamon, Gingko Biloba, Omega 3 fish or flax oils, Chromium Picolinate, Licorice Root Tea, Vitamin E, Selenium and CoQ10.
– Linda Page, N.D., Ph.D., "Healthy Healing"

We all grow healthier in nature, gentle sunshine and love!
– Patricia Bragg

B-Vitamins Important for Healthy Heart

Evidence shows that certain B-vitamins help reduce the risk of heart disease by lowering the harmful amino acid *homocysteine* from the blood. Too much homocysteine brings damage to the cells lining blood vessel walls. A Harvard study shows that B-vitamins (B1, B3 *niacin*, B5 *pantothenic acid*, B6, B12 and folic acid) help reduce homocysteine levels in the blood. This is especially important for those who are at risk for cardiovascular problems, because 1 in every 3 people with cardiovascular disease have dangerously high levels of homocysteine.

Plant foods are major sources of vitamin B6 and folic acid. However, vitamin B12 is not found in vegetables. Vegetarians can obtain sufficient B12 from tofu, eggs (not more than 4 times weekly), fortified almond milk, plant based meats, Cremini mushrooms and seaweed or from vitamin supplements. We recommend a good quality nutritional yeast – a delicious flavor enhancer, rich in B-vitamins (even B12). We sprinkle it over salads, soups, veggies, potatoes, rice, beans, and popcorn. See our delicious popcorn recipe on page 150.

214

Niacin & Folic Acid Helps Protect the Blood

Folic acid plays a vital role in the smooth functioning of a healthy body. Revered as a brain food, it's needed for growth of red and white blood cells and the body's energy production. Deficiencies of folic acid, B6 and B12 can lead to serious conditions such as depression, insomnia, immune system problems and dangerously high homocysteine levels.

In addition to supplements, folic acid is found in dates, dark leafy greens, avocado, broccoli, citrus fruits, beans, peas and lentils (see more on list next page). Folic acid works best taken with vitamin C, B6 and B12.

There is strong evidence from over 200 studies that increased consumption of Folic Acid (from foods or supplements) helps prevent cardiovascular disease.
– Godfrey Oakley, M.D., Research Professor of Epidemiology at Emory University

What you focus on – you manifest in your life!

Healthy Food Sources of Folic Acid
– The Health Nutrient Bible, Lynn Sonberg

Food Source	mgs
Spinach, (raw or steamed) 1 Cup	262
Asparagus, (raw or steamed) 1 Cup	176
Lima beans, (raw or steamed) 1 Cup	156
Broccoli, (raw or steamed) 1 Cup	108
Wheat germ, 1/4 Cup	106
Beets, (raw or steamed) 1 Cup	90
Cauliflower, (raw or steamed) 1 Cup	64
Orange (navel), 1 medium	47
Cantaloupe, 1/2 melon	46
Cabbage, (raw or steamed) 1 Cup	40
Tofu, firm 1/2 Cup	37

Other healthy sources of Folic Acid are: green leafy vegetables, dates, black-eyed peas, sunflower seeds, kidney beans, and winter squash

Research has shown Niacin (B3) has the ability to lower LDL (bad cholesterol), raise HDL (good cholesterol), and lower triglyceride levels. It has been shown to provide better heart healthy protection than some statins.

215

Vitamin C is for Capillaries and Cholesterol

For your capillary health, turn to vitamin C. Thousands of studies conclude vitamin C makes healthier capillaries by reducing clotting in the bloodstream. Remember, your blood must move along your capillaries in single file, cell by cell. A blood clot can completely stop the flow of blood through these microscopic vessels! Researchers attribute other cardiovascular benefits to C, including clearing of cholesterol and calcium from arterial walls. It's a strong weapon against the hardening and clogging of your arteries. Taken before bedtime, studies show it prevents heart attacks during sleep and in the morning. This new information supports studies conducted over 40 years ago by pioneering Doctor G. C. Willis, whose patients showed improvements of arteriosclerosis in leg arteries when given 500 mg. vitamin C, 3 times daily. We daily get at least 3,000 mg. of mixed vitamin C (with rutin and bioflavonoids) and Quercetin in supplements and fresh citrus fruits, green leafy vegetables, tomatoes and in the many fruits and vegetables we eat.

Sunshine Vitamin D3 – Essential for Health

Vital vitamin D3 is a natural hormone and like other hormones it's manufactured in the body. It helps the body utilize calcium and phosphorus to build bones and teeth. Vitamin D3 also helps the skin heal and boosts your immune system. Statistics from a California survey of American women found those women with higher sun exposure and with a high dietary intake of vitamin D3, had a lower risk of breast cancer. Evidence also points to a link between vitamin D3 and reduced risk of colon cancer and bone fractures.

There is evidence supporting the near-miraculous healing power of Vitamin D3, a nutrient that is available free just by enjoying gentle sunlight on your skin. Small amounts of gentle sunlight on your skin cells cause them to manufacture vitamin D3. Even as little as 10 to 15 minutes, 2 to 3 times a week should be sufficient to meet your needs. Sunscreen can reduce or even shut down the synthesis of vitamin D3, so we recommend exposure to gentle early morning or late afternoon rays without use of sunscreen. People under 50 years need 1,000 IUs, 50-70 years need 2,000 IUs and those over 70 need 2,000-5,000 IUs of vitamin D3 daily, more in special cases. Older people's ability to produce vitamin D3 from sunlight declines. That's why it's important for those over 70 to get vitamin D3 from supplements and foods: wheat germ, raw sunflower seeds, cod liver oil, sweet potatoes, corn bread, eggs, alfalfa, saltwater fish, sardines, salmon, tuna, liver and natural vegetable oils are good sources of vitamin D3.

An analysis of more that 15,000 Americans, those with low blood levels of Vitamin D3, were 30% more likely to have high blood pressure, 40% more apt to have high triglycerides, 98% more likely to be diabetic and 129% more apt to be obese. Researchers noted that low Vitamin D3 may also be a culprit for Fibromyalgia, Multiple Sclerosis, Rheumatoid Arthritis and other joint diseases.

Vitamin D3 is major protective factor guarding against chemical sensitivities and infections. Cod liver oil which parents once gave automatically to children is an excellent preventive medicine, with high concentrations of vitamins A and D3.
– Dr. Michael Schachter, Columbia University

Five Ways Vitamin D3 Can Save Your Life

1. **Reduces Risk of Heart Disease:** Vitamin D3 improves blood flow by relaxing the blood vessels and lowering blood pressure.

2. **Promotes Weight Loss:** You need Vitamin D3 to effectively help you lose weight. Your insulin works better and Vitamin D3 helps you lose belly fat. Diabetes is also related to low Vitamin D3 levels.

3. **Helps reduce Risk of Early, Premature Death**.

4. **Fewer Bone Fractures**: Without Vitamin D3, calcium can't be absorbed. But if you get enough vitamin D3, it helps you avoid osteoporosis, bone fractures and falling, which are causes of morbidity among elderly.

5. **Helps Fight Cancer:** D3 improves the functioning of your immune system that helps fight cancer.

Five Ways To Get Vitamin D3

1. **15 minutes of high-noon sun exposure** in warmer climates a few times a week. *(We prefer early or late sun.)*

2. **Fatty Fish and Cod Liver Oil:** If you have been warned to stay out of the sun, another good source of Vitamin D3 is oily fish, such as salmon, tuna, mackerel and trout.

3. **Fortified Dairy Products** (*We prefer non-dairy.*)

4. **Multi-Vitamin Supplements**: Most all multi-vitamins have a substantial amount of vitamin D3.

5. **Vitamin D3 Supplements:** 1000 to 2000 of IUs Vitamin D3 daily are recommended. (*Seniors 2000 to 3000 IUs.*)

Taken from: "Good Morning America's"
Medical Contributor Marie Savard

Vitamin D3 is made when UVB light from the sun is absorbed by the skin. This is the most natural form. Most supplements sold today are Vitamin D3 (animal source – lanolin) or Vitamin D2 (fungus/yeast derived) ideal for vegetarians/ vegans. Vitamin D3 is the more potent form of Vitamin D and has a better stable shelf-life. – Learn more by reading "The Vitamin D Solution" by Michael Holick, Ph.D., M.D. Professor of Boston University, recipient of prestigious "Linus Pauling Prize" for his extensive research on Vitamin D.

Morning light helps best in regulation of body's circadian rhythm and energy balance. Circadian rhythm is the body's physical, mental and behavioral changes that follow a roughly 24-hour cycle.

Vitamin E – Essential For Heart Health

According to Canada's Pioneer Shute brothers and scientist Dr. Richard Passwater, we all need vitamin E for the general health and proper body functioning. It's an essential vitamin for cardiovascular health. A low vitamin E level in the blood is one of the most reliable warning indicators of heart disease risk and future cardiovascular problems.

Why is vitamin E essential? It prevents damage by free radicals formed when fat is exposed to oxygen and heat. Vitamin E protects the arteries by neutralizing oxidized cholesterol. It helps prevent the red blood cells from clumping together, dissolves blood clots and increases oxygenation of blood, which improves the heart's supply of oxygen. Vitamin E dilates the capillaries, improves capillary strength and helps protect against cardiovascular scarring after a heart attack! It also helps provide relief from complaints of poor circulation, like leg cramps, cold feet and hands. We recommend a daily allowance of 400 to 800 IU's of natural mixed-tocopherol. In addition to supplements, there are significant quantities of vitamin E in wheat germ, cold-pressed vegetable oils, organic whole grains, dark leafy green vegetables, beans, raw nuts and seeds and our favorite, sunflower seeds.

E Tocotrienols: alpha, betta, gamma & delta

A study found that Vitamin E Tocotrienols lowered the damage to the heart muscle by 75%. These compounds demonstrate vitamin E-like activity, with great added protection benefits that help with serious heart problems. They help lower cholesterol and there's further evidence E Tocotrienols provide greater antioxidant protection against lipid peroxidation (cell damage) than standard vitamin E. People with metabolic syndrome run more than twice the risk of developing cardiovascular disease and diabetes. Researchers found "tocotrienols" improved lipid profiles and helped reduce atherosclerotic lesions, decreased blood glucose and normalized blood pressure. E Tocotrienols can be purchased in health stores as a single supplement – or as part of vitamin E with mixed E Tocopherols.

Vitamin E-Rich Healthy Foods Are Important for Healthy Hearts

Here's a list of healthy foods that contain the following notable amounts of precious vitamin E. Buy organic sources – they are best. Reference from *The National Institutes of Health*.

Food	Quantity	Vitamin E IU's
Apples	1 medium	1.21
Almonds	1/4 cup	13.37
Bananas	1 medium	0.40
Barley	1/2 cup	4.20
Beans, navy	1/2 cup	3.60
Bell Peppers	1 cup slices	0.94
Blueberries	1 cup	2.18
Broccoli	1 cup	1.12
Butter (salt-free)	6 tablespoons	2.40
Carrots	1 cup	0.45
Celery, green	1/2 cup	2.60
Corn oil	1 tablespoon	2.83
Eggs, fertile	2	2.62
Grapefruit	1/2	0.52
Kale	1/2 cup	8.00
Lettuce	6 leaves	0.50
Olive Oil (virgin)	1 Tbsp	2.38
Onions, raw	2 medium	0.26
Oranges	1 small	0.24
Papaya	1 medium	5.06
Peas, green	1 cup	4.00
Potatoes, white	1 medium	0.06
Potatoes, sweet	1 small	4.00
Rice, brown	1 cup cooked	2.40
Rye	1/2 cup	3.00
Soybean Oil	1 Tbsp	2.24
Sunflower Seeds, raw	1 oz.	8.94
Tomato	1 medium	1.01
Wheat Germ Oil	1 Tbsp	26.20

A study of nurses whose daily intake of Vitamin E was 800 IU's or more, yielded a 36% lower risk of heart attack and 23% lower risk of stroke!

Vitamin E protects cells from damaging effects of free radicals, which damage cells and might contribute to the development of heart disease and cancer. – ods.od.nih.gov

Vitamin E & Raw Wheat Germ – Health Builders

Mother Nature invested raw wheat germ with one of the most valuable nutrients – vitamin E. Now it is coming to the aid of civilized man to help him regain the robust health he lost by eating devitalized foods. In the flour milling process, refining removes the raw wheat germ to create white flour (the staff of death). Millers realize wheat germ is fragile and goes rancid quickly. Refined foods have a long shelf life. Many Americans demand things they buy never spoil! That is why many American foods are refined and over 700 chemicals and poisons are being used to preserve (embalm) them!

Dr. Cureton, often regarded as "The Father of Physical Fitness," who is recognized as one of the greatest authorities on internal and external physical fitness, recommended raw wheat germ, wheat germ oil and vitamin E capsules. They are especially useful in providing a great boost for athletes and others who desire to be in the highest state of physical fitness! Athletic coaches all over the world have followed this advice to get the best performance from their athletes. In our opinion *raw wheat germ (vacuum packed), wheat germ oil and Vitamin E should be part of the nutritional program of everyone* – not just athletes! Vitamin E capsules are also recommended as the oil is more protected from rancidity.

Wheat germ is a fantastic food that's available in flakes and coarse powder. We sprinkle it over raw garden salads, potatoes, vegetables, soups, etc. It has a pleasant, nutty taste. Don't forget you should refrigerate your wheat germ after you open it to keep it fresh.

Wheat germ contains 4.53 mg of vitamin E per 1 oz. serving, according to the United States Department of Agriculture's nutrient database. Wheat germ oil provides even more vitamin E per serving, with just 1 Tbsp. containing 20.3 mg. One tablespoon of wheat germ oil provides more than the recommended daily allowance of 15 mg of vitamin E. – www.LiveStrong.com

Vitamin E – dynamic weapon against wrinkles and ageing. – Prevention Magazine

Vitamin E helps prevent breakdown of body tissues.

Wheat germ helps to promote a healthy heart – it has good source of omega-3 fatty acids, which helps lower cholesterol and blood pressure.

Beta-Carotene Protects Against Heart Disease

Beta carotene plays an extremely important part in promoting heart health. More than 200 studies have confirmed that foods rich in flavonoids, carotenoids and other antioxidants can improve heart health, create a stronger immune system and reduce the risk of other health conditions. Beta-carotene is transformed in the body into vitamin A, which helps protect against heart disease in several ways. The most important is its ability to neutralize the toxic free radicals (see pages 28-30).

What is beta-carotene? Beta-carotene is probably the most well known of the carotenoids, a phytonutrients family (see page 139-141) that represents one of the most widespread groups of naturally occurring pigments. It is known as "pro-vitamin A" compound, able to convert into retinol, an active form of vitamin A. In recent years, beta-carotene has received a tremendous amount of attention as a potential anti-cancer and anti-ageing compound. Beta-carotene is a powerful antioxidant, protecting the cells of the body from damage caused by free radicals.

You should not take high-dose supplements of beta-carotene alone, but get it in combination with your diet. Food sources of beta-carotene include sweet potatoes, carrots, spinach, turnip greens, winter squash, collard greens, cilantro and fresh thyme. To maximize the availability of carotenoids in foods listed below, some should be eaten raw in salads, steamed lightly or baked.

Healthy Food Sources of Beta Carotene

Food Source	mcgs
Pumpkin – bake or steam (1 cup)	17,003
Sweet Potatoes – bake or steam (1 cup)	13,308
Carrots – fresh, slice or grate (1 cup)	10,605
Turnip greens – steam & drain (1 cup)	6,588
Kale – raw, chop (1 cup)	6,181
Butternut squash – raw, grate (1 cup)	5,916
Cantaloupe – fresh, dice (1 cup)	3,151
Spinach – raw, chop (1 cup)	1,688
Mango – fresh, dice (1 cup)	734
Apricot – fresh (1)	383

Magnesium For Your Heart, Blood & Arteries

Magnesium provides many benefits for your heart health. It reduces blood pressure and controls the skipping heart. It relaxes the muscles of the artery walls and improves blood flow. It's vital to your health and enzymatic activity. Magnesium helps shuttle potassium in and out of cells, maintaining proper membrane balance (homeostasis). It acts like a calcium channel blocker to stabilize cardiac conduction, heart muscle and vascular membranes. Please be alert to the vital importance of magnesium! It keeps your heart, blood and arteries working together!

Deficiencies in this essential mineral are often the root of many cardiovascular problems. A deficiency can interfere with the nerves and muscle impulses. Deficiencies can also produce all kinds of problems in the body – ranging from heart problems, dental decay and osteoporosis to muscular cramping, hyperactivity, muscular twitches, poor sleep patterns and excessive frequency or uncontrolled urination patterns. Side-effects can lead to high blood pressure, cardiac arrhythmia, cardiac arrest and stress damage in arterial walls! Despite dietary sources many adults and children living in so-called civilized cultures have low levels of this essential mineral in their bodies. This is due to leeching caused by coffee, tea, cola, carbonated beverages and the ravages of long-term bad diets containing refined sugars, toxic aspartame and other sweets! Also junk fast foods made from refined flours and foods containing high fat, high sugar, high salt and high cholesterol foods.

Though magnesium naturally occurs in most raw foods, a healthy daily amount of 250 mg. is hard to attain eating processed foods. **Rich in magnesium are: organic apples, apricots, avocados, bananas, green leafy vegetables, garlic, beans, raw nuts and seeds, brown rice, tofu, whole wheat and other whole grains.** Herbs such as cayenne, alfalfa, fennel, hops, paprika and others add magnesium for heart health! (See web: *all-natural.com*)

Magnesium is a superstar nutrient that plays a role in approximately 300 functions in the body. – Life Extension Magazine • www.lef.org

222

Calcium: The Other Half of the Dynamic Duo

Calcium is important too, because of its synergistic relationship with magnesium! Consider a shocking fact that 85% of Americans are deficient in calcium! Most people associate calcium with teeth and bones, which is correct since a deficiency of this important mineral will lead to deterioration of these hard tissues. Calcium is also very important for the nerves of the body. Many people suffer leg cramps due to calcium deficiency. Calcium also plays an important role in heart functioning. Calcium is a natural constituent of the material that causes blood to clot. If we don't have calcium in our blood, we could prick a finger with a needle and bleed to death! Low levels of calcium can increase your vulnerability to high blood pressure. But be cautious about how much calcium you take. Recommended Daily Amount is 1,000 mg. with 500 mg magnesium. More than 2,000 mg of calcium daily could cause kidneys to excrete magnesium!

Every few minutes the heart is bathed by the calcium of the body chemistry. It is a crucial component in the activity of a healthy heart. Being the most powerful muscle in the entire body, the heart requires adequate calcium for its efficient functioning. Be good to your heart and maintain a good calcium balance. Study calcium chart below.

Calcium Content of Some Common Foods

Food Source	mgs	Food Source	mgs
Almonds, 1 oz	80	Kale, (raw/steamed)	180
Artichokes, (raw/steamed)	51	Kohlrabi, (raw/steamed)	40
Beans, (kidney, pinto, red)	89	Mustard greens, 1 cup	138
Beans, (great northern, navy)	128	Oatmeal, 1 cup	120
Beans, (white)	161	Orange, 1 large	96
Blackstrap molasses, 1 Tbsp	137	Prunes, 4 whole	45
Bok choy, (raw/steamed)	158	Raisins, 4 oz.	45
Broccoli, (raw/steamed)	178	Rhubarb, (cooked) 1 cup	105
Brussels sprouts, (raw/steamed)	56	Rutabaga, (raw/steamed)	72
Buckwheat pancake	99	Sesame seeds (unhulled) 1 oz	381
Cabbage, (raw/steamed)	50	Spinach (raw/steamed)	244
Cauliflower, (raw/steamed)	34	Soybeans,	73
Collards, (raw/steamed)	152	Soymilk, fortified	150
Corn tortilla	60	Tofu, firm	258
Cornbread, 1 piece	28	Turnip greens, 1 cup	198
Figs, (5 medium)	135	Whole wheat bread, 1 slice	17

Sources: "Back to Eden", Jethro Kloss; "Health Nutrient Bible", Lynn Sonberg; website: vrg.org/nutrition/calcium.htm, chart by Brenda Davis, R.D.

Milk is Not a Good Source of Calcium

Nearly everyone has the idea that the problem of calcium deficiency will be solved if they just drink milk. This is not completely true. In the first place, practically all the milk in the U.S. is pasteurized, which robs and greatly reduces the availability of milk's calcium. (*NotMilk.com*)

Dr. Harold D. Lynch – famous author, researcher and physician – said, *"the use of milk as a beverage has added more complications than benefits to child nutrition."* He further stated, *"milk may often be a primary cause of poor nutrition in children!"*

Most All Natural Foods Rich in Calcium

There are some very fine sources of calcium other than milk! Scientists feel raw bonemeal is one of the best sources, as well as eggshell calcium, oyster shell calcium and bone marrow calcium. We prefer the calcium found in kale, spinach, corn, beans, veggies, tofu and sesame seeds – see chart on previous page. In fact, as Dr. Lynch and Dr. Neal Barnard point out, all natural foods contain appreciable amounts of important calcium.

(224)

Read 2 important books on milk and why it's best to avoid:

- *Mad Cows and Milk Gate* by Virgil Hulse, M.D.
- *Milk, the Deadly Poison* by Robert Cohen

Also visit these websites:

- *www.NotMilk.com*
- *pcrm.org* (Physicians Committee for Responsible Medicine)

Many osteoporosis studies consistently conclude that vegetarians have stronger bones than meat-eaters. Many studies show that it's healthier to avoid meat and dairy products for optimum heart health.

For optimal bone and cardiovascular health, nutritional experts for the past 40 years have urged those who take calcium to also supplement with magnesium, vitamin D and K. – Life Extension Magazine, visit: www.lef.org.

Take 1,000 mg calcium daily in conjunction with 500 mg magnesium daily. Postmenopausal women are advised to take 1,500 mg calcium. Choose a calcium formula that contains mixed compounds such as citrate, carbonate, aspartate and gluconate in combination with similar magnesium complex.

For arrhythmia, magnesium orotate works miracles, along with calcium.

Locations in the Body Where Osteoporosis, Arthritis, Pain and Misery Hit the Hardest

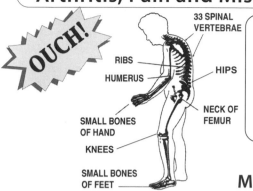

OSTEOPOROSIS
Affects over 60 Million and Kills 400,000 Americans Annually
Estimated 50% of adults 65 years or older also suffer from Arthritis.

Boron: Miracle Trace Mineral For Healthy Bones

BORON – An important trace mineral for healthier and stronger bones that also helps the body absorb more vital calcium, minerals and necessary hormones! Good boron sources are most organic veggies, fresh and sun-dried fruits, avocados, prunes, and raw nuts.

The U.S. Dept. of Agriculture's Nutrition Lab in Grand Forks, ND, says Boron is usually found in soil and foods, but many Americans eat a diet low in Boron. They conducted a 17 week study which showed a daily 3 to 6 mgs. Boron supplement enabled participants to reduce loss (demineralization) of calcium, phosphorus and magnesium from their bodies. This loss is usually caused by eating processed fast foods, drinking tap waters (distilled is best), eating lots of meat, salt, sugar and fat and a dietary lack of fresh vegetables, fruits and whole grains. *(all-natural.com)*

225

Scientific studies show women benefit from a healthy lifestyle that includes vitamin D3 sunshine and exercise (even weight-lifting) to maintain healthier bones, combined with distilled water, low-fat, high-fiber, carbohydrates, and fresh organic fruits, salads, sprouts, greens and vegetable diet. This lifestyle helps protect against heart disease, high blood pressure, cancer and many other ailments! I'm happy to see science now agrees with my Dad who first stated these health truths in the 1920's.

For more hormone and osteoporosis facts read pioneer Dr. John R. Lee's book –
"What Your Doctor May Not Tell You About Menopause"

Boron helps keep skeletal structure strong by adding to bone density, preventing Osteoporosis, treating Arthritis and improving strength and muscle mass. Boron helps facilitate calcium directly into the bones. Boron protects bones by regulating Estrogen function. Boron is naturally found in beans, nuts, avocados, berries, plums, oranges and grapes. Boron helps relieve menopause symptoms and PMS. – Dr. Axe

Potassium Helps Strengthen the Heart

The heart is a large muscular organ and your master pump. It uses large amounts of potassium to keep going strong and healthy, hour after hour, for your entire life! It is the hardest working organ in the body. The heart must have a constant, continuous supply of power and energy to continue beating! Apple cider vinegar contains natural potassium that combines with healthy heart foods to make the heart muscle stronger and also help to normalize blood pressure and cholesterol.

Take an extra 1 tsp. of raw organic apple cider vinegar (ACV) in 1/2 glass distilled/purified water, twice daily between meals – good before exercise. But also enjoy your basic 3 ACV drinks daily (see pages 150).

Potassium is the Master Mineral

Potassium is an essential mineral for the body because it puts toxic poisons in solution so they can be flushed out of the body. **The body is self-cleansing, self-correcting, self-repairing and self-healing!** Just give it the tools to work with and you will have a painless, tireless, ageless body, regardless of age! Forget calendar years, for age is not toxic! You age prematurely when you suffer from potassium deficiencies and malnutrition! This low Vital Force and waste buildup (poor elimination) allows disease to proliferate.

The Bragg Healthy Lifestyle helps you rebuild your Vital Force. Watch the transformation that takes place in your body when you faithfully follow the ACV regime. You can, and will become the kind of person you want to be! It's exciting to plan, plot and follow through!

Please follow this program closely, don't try to do everything listed here immediately! Remember, it took you a long time of living by wrong habits to cause any of the problems your body might have now. So, it's going to take time for the body to cleanse, repair and rebuild itself into a more *perfect health home* for you! Please remember, *your body is your temple while on this earth – so cherish it and protect it!*

Health Basics of Essential Fatty Acids (EFA)

Adequate intake of EFA results in numerous health benefits – prevention of atherosclerosis, reduced incidence of heart disease and stroke, and relief from symptoms associated with ulcerative colitis, menstrual and joint pain.

Omega-3 and omega-6 essential fatty acids (EFA) are vital components of cell membranes. The omega-3 fatty acid, found in fish oil, is important for patients with heart disease. This fatty acid can affect the body's immune system, inflammatory response, blood flow, blood pressure and blood coagulability. Omega-3 fatty acids can have a marked effect on reducing the triglyceride levels.

It is also important to consume these fatty acids in the proper ratio. Omega-6s compete with omega-3s for use in the body, and therefore excessive intake of omega-6 can inhibit omega-3. Ideally, the ratio of omega-6 to omega-3 should be between 1:1 and 4:1. Unfortunately, Americans consume these fatty acids at the wrong ratio and are consequently unable to reap the benefits of omega-3s. This imbalance is due to processed foods and oils, which are now common in the Western diet. To combat this issue it is necessary to eat a low-fat diet with minimal processed foods and with naturally occurring omega-3 fatty acids. (see *pcrm.org*)

Studies confirm omega-3 fatty acids in fish and flax oil provide tremendous protection from heart disease. They aid in the stabilization of the heart's electrical activity reducing the risk of fatal arrhythmias and sudden cardiac death. Almost all fresh, raw, unprocessed nuts, grains and seeds contain substantial quantities of the omega-6 fatty acids. Fish oil and flaxseed are the most abundant sources of omega-3 fatty acids.

WORLD'S HEALTHIEST FOODS RICH IN OMEGA-3 FATS

FOOD	% Daily Value	FOOD	% Daily Value
Flaxseeds	133%	Brussels Sprouts	11%
Walnut	113%	Winter Squash	8%
Chia Seeds	102%	Broccoli	8%
Soybeans	43%	Spinach	7%

Getting flax in your diet is important as brushing your teeth. Oil from flax seeds has highest proportion Omega-3 of any plant known. Flax and Chia seeds work as well as fish oil when it comes to lowering triglycerides and LDL cholesterol levels, while raising good HDL cholesterol. – Dr. David Williams

Great Sources of Omega-3 Fatty Acids

Plants: spinach, winter squash, broccoli, beans, walnuts.
Oils: flaxseed, chia seeds, olive oil, and walnut.
Seafood: salmon, tuna, sardines, anchovies and trout.

L-Arginine – Essential to Heart Health

L-Arginine is an amino acid that has shown promise in prevention of atherosclerosis. It is thought to be the primary source for production of nitrogen molecules involved in maintaining elasticity of blood vessels. Research has shown that L-Arginine may be helpful for people with high cholesterol.

Ubiquinol CoQ10 Combats Heart Disease, Cancer, Gum Disease and Ageing

Ubiquinol Coenzyme Q10, a potent important antioxidant that protects cells from free radicals, also is involved in energy production in cells. Although made by every body cell, production diminishes with age and disease.

The heart is one of the few body organs to function continuously without resting; therefore, the heart muscle requires the highest energetic support! Any condition that causes a decrease in CoQ10 could impair the heart's energetic capacity, thus leaving heart tissues more susceptible to free radical attack! In long term studies, Ubiquinol CoQ10 was found to prolong life by years, (100 mg. am and 50 mg. early evening). Cardiologist, Dr. Peter H. Langsjoen's co-authored study found patients reduced heart and blood pressure medications by 40-50% and 25% of patients became drug-free. (web: *lef.org*)

To increase your omega-3 intake try flaxseeds and chia seeds (page 131) and walnuts. 1/4 cup flaxseeds contains about 7 grams of omega-3, while 1/4 cup of walnuts contains about 2.3 grams. Add this nut-seed combination to salads, baked potatoes, trail mix, granola, etc. Other omega-3 sources include: fish and olive oil – don't hi-fry, only lightly sauté. Add 2 Tbsps flaxseeds (ground) daily to foods, to be closer to the recommended 4 grams of omega-3.

CoEnzyme Q10 (CoQ10) is a vitamin-like substance produced by the body that's necessary for proper functioning of our cells. CoQ10 levels decrease with age and has been found to be low in people with chronic diseases, including Parkinson's disease, cancer, diabetes, and chronic heart conditions. Studies show routine use of CoQ10 supplements for muscle pain associated with statins helps reduce pain!

Oligomeric Proanthocyanidins (OPCs)

You've probably heard about the benefits of red wine, green tea (caffeine free), and grape juice. All are in the family of oligomeric proanthocyanidins (OPCs). OPCs are flavonoid complexes, found in most plants and a part of the human diet. They are found in large quantities in grape seed extract and grape skins, in red grapes, in the red skins of peanuts, in coconuts and apples. These free radical scavengers are quickly absorbed into the bloodstream where they cross the blood/brain barrier. OPCs may help protect against the effects of internal and environmental stresses such as cigarette smoking and pollution, as well as supporting normal body metabolic processes. Looking at some of the benefits linked to OPCs is like looking at a shopping list for a long and healthy life. Let us list just some of the amazing discoveries about this simple wonder nutrient. OPCs have been shown to:

- Prevent oxidation of LDL "bad" cholesterol, thereby lowering your risk of cardiovascular disease
- Reduce cholesterol plaque buildup on blood vessel walls
- Decrease blood stickiness, thus excessive blood clotting
- Increase the strength and elasticity of capillaries, improving vascular function
- Reduce swelling, inflammation, degeneration of veins, and edema, helping to prevent circulation problems and varicose veins
- Improve blood vessel elasticity and lower blood pressure
- Protect against many types of eye conditions including diabetic retinopathy (the most common cause of blindness in diabetics), cataracts and glaucoma
- Decrease discomfort associated with menopause and premenstrual syndrome

If you're not already convinced that OPCs are a combination healer and fountain of youth, let us tell you that OPCs have also been linked to fighting chronic fatigue, arthritis, allergies, Alzheimer's disease, as well as other degenerative diseases. Grapeseed extract and pinebark extract are great ways to get your daily dose of OPCs. We recommend 30-60 mg daily. See front inside cover for more info.

THE MIRACLES OF APPLE CIDER VINEGAR FOR A STRONGER, LONGER, HEALTHIER LIFE

> *The old adage is true:*
> *"An apple a day keeps the doctor away."*

- Helps promote a youthful skin and vibrant healthy body
- Helps remove artery plaque, infections and body toxins
- Helps fight germs, viruses, bacteria and mold naturally
- Helps retard old age onset in humans, pets and farm animals
- Helps regulate calcium metabolism
- Helps keep blood the right consistency
- Helps regulate women's menstruation, relieves PMS, and UTI
- Helps normalize urine pH, relieving frequent urge to urinate
- Helps digestion, assimilation and helps balances the pH
- Helps protect against food poisoning and even brings relief if you do get it
- Helps relieve sore throats, laryngitis and throat tickles and cleans out throat mucus and gum toxins
- Helps detox the body so sinus, asthma and flu sufferers can breathe easier and more normally
- Helps banish acne, athlete's foot, soothes burns, sunburns
- Helps prevent itching scalp, dandruff, and dry hair
- Helps fight arthritis and helps remove crystals and toxins from joints, tissues, organs and entire body
- Helps control and normalize body weight

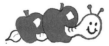

– Paul C. Bragg, ND, PhD., Health Crusader, Originator of Health Stores

Our sincere blessings to you, dear friends, who make our lives so worthwhile and fulfilled by reading our teachings on natural living as our Creator laid down for us to follow. He wants us to follow the simple path of natural living. This is what we teach in our books and health crusades worldwide. Our prayers reach out to you and your loved ones for the best in health and happiness. We must follow the laws He has laid down for us, so we can reap this precious health physically, mentally, emotionally and spiritually!

HAVE AN APPLE HEALTHY LIFE!

With Love,

Organic Raw Unfiltered Apple Cider Vinegar with the "Mother" is #1 food I recommend to stop heartburn, gerd, gas, indigestion and for maintaining body's vital acid-alkaline balance and digestion. – Gabriel Cousens, M.D., Author, "Conscious Eating"

Chapter 23

Heart Healthy Programs

While outlining our Healthy Heart Fitness Program we have told you in detail about the vicious enemies of the heart. Know your enemies and keep away from them! If you have lived a haphazard life and have damaged your heart, we believe that you can still make a comeback and build a healthy heart for yourself. Remember that your body is self-cleansing, self-repairing and self-healing! Given the chance, it will do its best to rebuild a vigorous heart for you. But you must work with your body – not against it!

Do not be discouraged if you have an ailing or damaged heart. Faithfully following our program of clean, natural living will help you to live out your natural life span! Yes, your miraculous body possesses tremendous recuperative powers which – if fully used – are of great help even in the most serious cases of heart trouble.

Bragg Healthy Heart Fitness Pointers

 231

💜 **A vegetarian diet is healthier.** Instead of meat, eat unsaturated vegetarian proteins – such as tofu, beans, raw seeds and nuts such as: sunflower, sesame, flaxseed, pumpkin, almonds, pecans, and walnuts.

💜 **Use no refined salt** – toss the salt shaker! (Use coconut aminos, garlic, onions, fresh herbs, lemon or sea kelp.)

💜 **Eat no dairy products** – milk, cheese, butter – high in clogging, saturated fats (use almond or rice milk.)

💜 **If you want to eat eggs, limit it to 4 a week.** Organically fed, free-range chicken eggs are healthiest.

💜 **Fruits and vegetables – organic, raw or lightly steamed or cooked** – should form 60% to 70% of your diet.

💜 **Don't use any white sugars or toxic commercial substitutes** such as aspartame, NutraSweet, etc. – they contain harmful chemicals (see page 70-71).

💜 **Fast for a 24-hour period weekly** (pages 163-170). This gives your heart and vital organs physiological rest. It also helps reduce cholesterol and toxins in the body and arteries.

💜 **A low-fat diet, ample exercise and brisk walking with deep breathing** help keep cholesterol levels normal.

Bragg Healthy Heart Program:

- **Absolutely NO SMOKING!** (see pages 84-88)
- **Get plenty of recharging sleep.** (pages 171-176)
- **Don't let anything put undue pressure** on you. Worry, stress, and tension do not necessarily cause a heart attack – but they don't help you avoid it either!
- **Eat healthy, simple, natural, organic foods and products and please don't over-eat.** (see pages 136-138)
- **Eat slowly – chew your food thoroughly.** Chewing is first process in digestion. Saying grace helps digestion!
- **Get plenty of regular exercise.** Although complete rest may be necessary just after an acute heart attack or when the heart is very weak. When this stage is past you will find regular daily exercise a great help in rebuilding and revitalizing the heart and circulation. (see pages 89-98)
- **Don't get into emotional arguments,** they waste precious nervous energy! Walk away from unpleasant people – it's best to avoid them completely!
- **Get into the Happiness Habit!** A cheerful, happy disposition helps promote health and longevity.
- **Stay away from all artificial stimulants and sweeteners** – coffee, tea (caffeine), soda/cola and alcohol. Also no Aspartame and chemical sugar substitutes.
- **Briskly Walk Daily! Breathe deeply!** (see pages 90-93)

232

Following Bragg's Heart Fitness Program

Would you trust the repair of your car to someone who had no knowledge of automobiles? Of course not! It is never too late to obtain and apply health knowledge. We have already described to you the structure and functioning of your precious heart and circulatory system and explained the importance of keeping the blood cholesterol at a healthy normal level. We suggest that you reread this book from time to time. Let this Program be your Faithful Guide on the Highway to Super Health.

Stress and emotional turmoil can cause or worsen high blood pressure. Reduce stress through regular exercise, which should be a part of your lifestyle, to lower blood pressure and improve heart health. – Health & Nutrition Breakthrough

Mother Nature cannot be rushed – but if you cooperate with her, you can have *the heart of a lion*. If you have a weak heart or weak *pipes* that are clogged, remember that it took a long time to get them into that condition. Be patient with Mother Nature while the regeneration, rejuvenation and cleansing processes take place within your body.

A fit, youthful heart can be yours, if you are willing to work for it! No one else can make your heart strong. It depends entirely on you. Your eating habits, your daily lifestyle and your physical activity will determine the condition of your heart and the health you will enjoy.

Dr. John Harvey Kellogg's Famous Vegetarian Diet for Heart Patients

Dr. John Harvey Kellogg was the founder and director of the great Battle Creek Sanitarium at Battle Creek, Michigan. Sick people from all over the world – even royalty – traveled there to be under his personal care. My father was fortunate enough to work with him.

As soon as a heart attack victim was brought to the Sanitarium, Dr. Kellogg would put them on a strict vegetarian diet with the advice that this should be a lifetime diet. It was a strict, exclusively vegetarian regime consisting of fruit, vegetables, seeds and nuts. No meat, no fish, no eggs, no dairy products, no coffee, no alcohol and no salt were allowed. Dr. Kellogg believed this strict vegetarian diet was the only one which a heart sufferer should eat because it contained absolutely no cholesterol. It was also a salt-free diet. The only drinks allowed were herb teas, fresh fruit and vegetable juices and distilled water. Dr. Kellogg told Dad that people who had come to him with serious heart damage had lived as many as 50 additional years on this strict vegetarian diet.

Dr. Kellogg himself lived and practiced until he was into his 90's He was a strict lacto-vegetarian, eating only a small amount of natural cheese and 3 eggs weekly with the otherwise completely vegetarian diet which he advocated for his heart patients. Today a great many doctors and nutritionists have joined him in recommending a vegetarian diet for all heart patients. See the following pages for Dr. Kellogg's menu ideas.

Dr. Kellogg's Famous Menus:

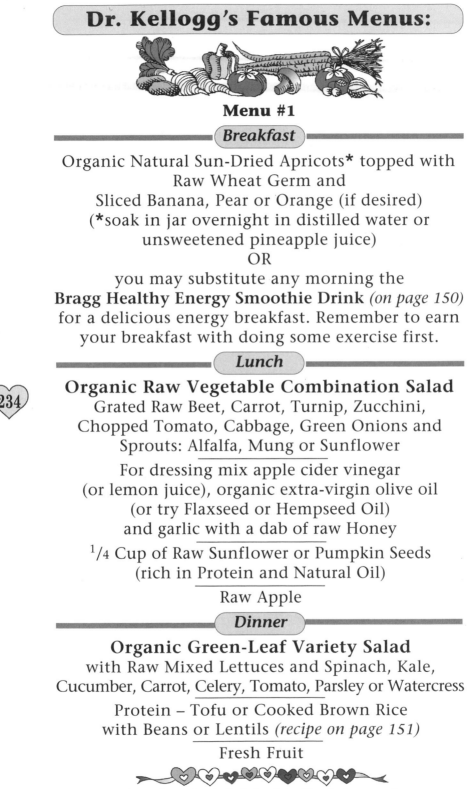

Menu #1

Breakfast

Organic Natural Sun-Dried Apricots* topped with
Raw Wheat Germ and
Sliced Banana, Pear or Orange (if desired)
(*soak in jar overnight in distilled water or
unsweetened pineapple juice)
OR
you may substitute any morning the
Bragg Healthy Energy Smoothie Drink *(on page 150)*
for a delicious energy breakfast. Remember to earn
your breakfast with doing some exercise first.

Lunch

Organic Raw Vegetable Combination Salad
Grated Raw Beet, Carrot, Turnip, Zucchini,
Chopped Tomato, Cabbage, Green Onions and
Sprouts: Alfalfa, Mung or Sunflower

For dressing mix apple cider vinegar
(or lemon juice), organic extra-virgin olive oil
(or try Flaxseed or Hempseed Oil)
and garlic with a dab of raw Honey

$1/4$ Cup of Raw Sunflower or Pumpkin Seeds
(rich in Protein and Natural Oil)

Raw Apple

Dinner

Organic Green-Leaf Variety Salad
with Raw Mixed Lettuces and Spinach, Kale,
Cucumber, Carrot, Celery, Tomato, Parsley or Watercress

Protein – Tofu or Cooked Brown Rice
with Beans or Lentils *(recipe on page 151)*

Fresh Fruit

Organic apples daily helps keep the doctor away!

234

Dr. Kellogg's Famous Menus:

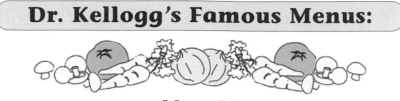

Menu #2

Breakfast

Apple Sauce*
Steel Cut Oats– hot cereal**
served with Honey, Blackstrap Molasses,
Pure Maple Syrup or Stevia (page 143)
100% Whole Wheat or Rye Toast
(*Make your own Apple Sauce, if desired add Honey)
(**Top and serve with Sliced Ripe Banana or other Fruit)

Lunch

Organic Raw Vegetable Combination Salad
(Same as 1st Day)
Vegetable Soup with Natural Barley and Lentils
Whole Rye Toast or Oat Bran-Raisin Muffin

Dinner

Cabbage, Apple & Carrot Coleslaw
with Spring Onions
Brown Rice or Baked Potato with Skin
Baked or Steamed Carrots and Peas
Fresh Fruit
OR
Avocado, Red Onion and Tomato Salad
Steamed Asparagus or Broccoli
Raw Nuts and Seeds of any kind
Fresh Fruit

*The greatest force in the human body is the natural drive of
the body to heal itself – but that force is not independent
of the belief system. Everything begins with belief.
What we believe is the most powerful option of all.
– Norman Cousins, author, "Anatomy of an Illness"*

*Studies show both beta carotene and vitamin C, abundantly found in fruits and
vegetables, play vital roles in preventing heart disease and cancers.*

"Abstinence and quietness – cure many diseases." – Hippocrates, 400 B.C.

Enjoy Positive Thinking and Positive Action

To have a healthy and powerful heart you must develop strong willpower. You must overcome all negative thoughts about the *inevitable* impacts that age supposedly ravages on the heart and body. Do not let cowards and weaklings influence you away from following this *Healthy Heart Fitness Program*! These fear mongers will try to impart their fear to you by telling you to go easy on exercise, fasting and life changes. Don't believe them! Have faith in your body's ability to improve!

When following this *Bragg Healthy Heart Fitness Program* and lifestyle you are working with Science and Mother Nature. Don't let unqualified people influence or deter you! Years of health research and investigation have gone into the development of this *Heart Fitness Program* in order to provide you with a master plan for building a strong, fit heart for a long, fulfilled, healthy life.

Six More Points to a Bragg Healthy Heart

236

We bring you this book not so much to help you as to help you help yourself! If we repeat certain points, it is with the zeal with which one taps a nail already driven home. Our main objective is to inspire you to a more intense enthusiasm for living The Bragg Healthy Lifestyle and to warn you against certain dangers which you may have easily overlooked. Throughout this book we have strongly stressed these six important points to faithfully follow:

1. You have but one heart and one life – you should faithfully take care of these priceless treasures!
2. Your body must obey the commands of your mind, for flesh needs a strong health captain!
3. Every bad habit that weakens your heart and shortens your life must be broken and then banished forever!
4. You should demand of yourself a higher living standard for more health, peace of mind and happiness!
5. You should regard your body (your temple) as you would a fine instrument or precision machine whose care and control is in your capable hands!
6. You must draw closer to Mother Nature so as to keep your life simple as 1, 2, 3 as your years increase!

Let us, then throw ourselves into her loving and understanding arms! Try to understand and follow these wise laws and live as Mother Nature wants us to live – in superb health for a long, active life of helping this world to be a better, safer, healthier place for us all.

Back-to-Nature is Always Best

The complete naturalist's healthy goal is to identify so completely with Mother Nature, that self and the world become one. To do this, keep your life simple as 1, 2, 3, filled with peace, joy and love. Then with serene, clear-eyed confidence put yourself into Mother Nature's hands to run your machine, heal your hurts and comfort you in sickness and adversity.

Let your body be nourished by natural food, pure distilled (rain) water, fresh air and gentle sunlight. Exercise and relax your body and let Mother Nature do the rest! Treat your body with the same care and wisdom that you would a champion animal. Surely as your animal will take prizes, so will you! Some sneer at health-minded, back-to-nature people. We who believe in Mother Nature enjoy enriched, happy, healthy lives!

Get Close to Mother Earth

It is good to establish contact with Mother Earth, her soil, water, air and sun. Let your bare feet grip into the soft grass or to feel soft mud or sand and squish it between your toes! We love gentle sun (before 10 a.m. or after 3 p.m.) and air baths with few clothes on. We love exercising, stretching, walking and swimming on the beach beside a sea, lake or river. Keep in close touch with Mother Earth, letting her strength and virtue pass into you through your skin and bare feet! *Modern living can complicate our lives with hot house living conditions!* Man was a healthier, happier creature when he lived simpler and closer to Mother Nature.

A healthy body is a guest-chamber for the soul and a sick body is a prison.
– Francis Bacon, English Lord Chancellor, Natural Philosopher (1561-1626)

Cheerfulness is the atmosphere in which all things thrive. – Jean Paul Richter

Follow the Laws of Mother Nature

In the past it was the middle-aged and older people who felt they had to seek drugs or other artificial means to hang onto life. Now, tragically, young people are using drugs of all kinds and throwing away their natural vitality, turning their backs on Mother Nature. Now our youth have become candidates for heart attacks. The heart is damaged by these stimulants and depressants.

The further we get away from living according to The Laws of Mother Nature, the sicker we get physically, mentally, emotionally and spiritually.

One of the dominant themes of this book is the idea that building a powerful heart at any age is a gradual return to a more natural form of living. Use natural healthy foods, vigorous exercise, deep breathing, restful sleeping, loose fitting clothing and enjoy the beautiful simplicity of life to reach a closeness to Mother Nature that makes you almost one with her! When you can feel the same strong, pure, elemental forces that manifest themselves in a pine tree expressing themselves in you, then you are on your way to positive, strong health principles.

Begin to live as Mother Nature wants you to live. Try to feel that she claims you and that you are part of all the glad and growing things on this Good Earth! Put yourself into Mother Nature's hands. We are all eager to aid you on the path to Supreme Health!

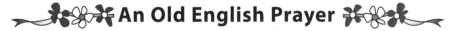

An Old English Prayer

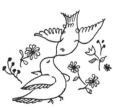

Give us Lord, a bit o' sun,
A bit o' work and a bit o' fun.
Give us in all the struggle and sputter,
Our daily bread and a bit of butter.
Give us health, our keep to make
And a bit to spare for others' sake.
Give us too, a bit of song,
And a tale and a book, to help us along.
Give us Lord, a chance to be
Our goodly best, brave, wise and free.
Our goodly best for ourselves and others,
'Til all men learn to live as brothers.

Dr. Linda Page's Healthy Heart Program*

Heart disease is still the biggest killer of Americans. A million of us die each year because of heart problems. Yet, most heart disease is 100% preventable with changes in diet and lifestyle. Natural Therapies have proven to reduce mortality better than aggressive medical intervention or even the most advanced drug treatment.

1. DIET & SUPER-FOODS Therapy

- **Your diet is your greatest asset in preventing heart disease.** A healthy heart diet has plenty of magnesium and potassium rich foods: fresh greens, sea foods and sea greens; flavonoids from pitted fruits, green herb teas, brown rice, whole grains, garlic and onions.

- **Reduce saturated fat to no more than 10% of your daily calorie intake.** Especially limit fats from animal sources and hydrogenated oils. Wisely pay conscious attention to avoiding red meats, caffeine products, refined sugars, fatty, salty and fried foods, prepared meats and soft drinks! The rewards are worth the effort.

239

- **Eat 70% of daily calories from complex carbohydrates like vegetables and grains; 20% from low fat protein sources.** Vitamin C-rich foods – tomatoes, citrus juice and apple cider vinegar greatly enhance iron absorption.

- **Eat less than 100mg per day of dietary cholesterol.** Keep cholesterol 180 and below (chart inside front cover).

- **Add 6 glasses of purified/distilled water daily** to your diet. It's the best diuretic for a healthy heart. (Chlorinated/ fluoridated water destroys vitamin E in the body.)

- **Blood Cleansing & Normalizing Herbs:** Burdock Root, Sarsaparilla, Chaparral, Ginger & Licorice Root, Alfalfa, Red Clover, Green Tea, Dandelion, Sea Greens, Yellow Dock Root, Hawthorn Berry, Chlorella and Barley Grass.

   Super foods for heart therapy are Aloe Vera Juice & Gel, herbs, royal jelly, bee pollen and Siberian Ginseng.

Super-foods are foods found in nature. They are low in calories and high in nutrients. They are superior sources of anti-oxidants and essential nutrients.

*Excerpts from "Healthy Healing" – by Linda Page

2. HERB & SUPPLEMENT Therapy

- **In an emergency:** 1 tsp. cayenne powder in water or juice or cayenne tincture (20 drops) in water, may help bring a person out of a heart attack; or take liquid Carnitine as directed. Also one-half dropperful Hawthorn extract every 15 minutes (see pages 212-213).

- **Tone the heart muscle:** CoQ10 with E Tocotrienols (helps lower cholesterol). Ascorbate with bioflavonoids, up to 5,000 mg daily. Evening Primrose Oil 1,000 mg 4 times daily. Magnesium rich herbs: Motherwort, Parsley or Magnesium 800 mg.

- **Improve blood flow:** Red Sage tea or Gingko Biloba extracts 2-3 times daily, Creatine 3,000 mg daily.

- **Antioxidants strengthen cardiovascular system and keep it clear:** Hawthorn & Grapeseed 100 mg 3x daily.

- **Boost your thyroid to reduce heart disease risk:** Spirulina, liquid chlorophyll, 2 Tbsp dry sea greens daily.

- **Cardiotonics help heart beat stronger and steadier:** CoQ10 60 mg 3x daily, Carnitine 1,000 mg daily, Cayenne-Ginger caps or garlic caps 6x daily, Siberian Ginseng caps 2,000 mg or tea 2 cups daily and wheat germ oil caps.

- **Phyto-estrogen heart protective herbs for women on menopause:** Ginkgo Biloba extract helps prevent ischemia-caused fibrillation. Vitex (chaste tree berry) Extract and Licorice Root Tea (delicious when fasting).

- **Heart disease preventives:** Folic Acid – B6 -100 mg & B12 - 2,500 mcg, helps keep down homocysteine levels.

- **Reduce blood stickiness to prevent heart attack:** Bromelain 1,500 mg regularly increases fibrinolysis Chromium picolinate, Omega-3 fish or flax oil 3 times daily.

- **To cleanse the arteries:** Vitamin E 800 IUs, Carnitine 1,000 mg and Lysine and Arginine 2,000 mg of each.

- **To help flush out infectious bacteria trapped in blocked lymph glands and blood vessels:** Echinacea and Goldenseal extract in combination.

240

Excerpts from "Healthy Healing" – by Linda Page

3. LIFESTYLE SUPPORT Therapy

- Bite down on tip of little finger to help stop a heart attack.
- Apply hot compresses and massage chest to ease heart attack.
- Take alternate hot /cold showers to increase circulation.
- Smoking constricts the arteries and can cause your blood pressure to skyrocket. Researchers estimate that 150,000 heart disease deaths could be prevented each year if Americans just quit smoking! Quit smoking now! (pg. 88)
- Do mild regular daily exercise (preferably brisk walking). Do deep breathing exercises daily for more body oxygen to stimulate your brain and to stay youthful with activity.
- Periodontal disease increases the chance of a heart attack by 2.7 times. Add CoQ10 – 100mg to your daily health program, good for teeth, gums and your heart!
- Add relaxation and a good daily laugh to your life. Also having a positive mental out-look does wonders for stress.

4. HEART REHABILITATION Program

This program is designed for those who have survived a heart attack or major heart surgery. Beginning and sticking to a new lifestyle that changes everything about the way you eat, exercise and handle stress, is a challenge. The following program is a blueprint you can use with confidence. It addresses main preventative needs – keeping your arteries clear and your blood slippery – goals that can be achieved through healthy diet and exercise.

- **Reduce saturated fats to 10% of your diet**; less if possible. Limit polyunsaturated oils to 10%. Add mono-unsaturates (olive oil, avocados, nuts and seeds). Add Essential Fatty Acids (fish, flax oil). Olive oil boosts healthy HDL-cholesterol levels and helps remove fats from blood.

Periodontal disease can lead to serious complications for those with coronary heart disease. It's the bacteria from the mouth that enters the bloodstream and attaches to fatty proteins in the blood vessels which may cause blood clots. Inflammation caused by periodontal disease may cause the arteries to harden. Brush your teeth, floss at lease twice daily and consult with your dentist.

*Excerpts from "Healthy Healing" – by Linda Page

- **Eat potassium-rich foods for cardiotonic activity:** spinach, chard, kale, broccoli, bananas, winter squash, sea greens, molasses, apricots, cantaloupe, papayas, sweet potatoes, mushrooms, tomatoes, carrot juice and yams.

- **Eat plenty of complex carbohydrates,** such as broccoli, peas, whole grain breads, vegetable pastas, potatoes, sprouts, tofu and brown rice. Have a green salad every day.

- **For essential omega-3 fatty acids,** have a couple of servings daily of walnuts, ground flaxseed or flaxseed oil.

- **Eat magnesium-rich foods for heart regulation:** tofu, wheat germ, oat or rice bran, broccoli, potatoes, lima beans, spinach, chard, bok choy and kale.

- **Eat high-fiber foods for a clean system and alkalinity:** whole grains, fruits and vegetables, legumes and herbs.

Almost all heart disease can be treated and prevented with improved nutrition. Refined, high fat, high calorie foods create heart problems. Natural, whole foods help relieve them! Full-fat dairy products like whole milk, ice cream and cheese are biggest dietary contributors to elevated LDL-cholesterol. Fried, salty, sugary foods, low-fiber, fatty and dairy foods, red meats, processed meats, tobacco and caffeine all contribute to clogged arteries, LDL bad cholesterol, high blood pressure and heart attacks!

Americans are in the highest risk category for heart disease. If you think conventional medicines will protect you, think again. Many experts think drug and surgical techniques to "protect" your heart are based on big bucks instead of health. Surgery alone cost Americans over $50 billion each year. Clearly, lives have been saved and extended, but drugs and surgery carry serious risks. Studies show that calcium channel blockers, the top selling blood pressure drugs, increase heart attack risk up to 60%. Many cholesterol-lowering statin drugs can cause serious liver toxicity, stomach distress and vision impairment. They also deplete CoQ10, an essential Coenzyme that strengthens the heart, by up to 50%.*

HERBS FOR CIRCULATORY STIMULATION: Dandelion, Alfalfa, Sea Greens, Yellow Dock Root, Chlorella, Hawthorn Berry, Marshmallow, Barley Grass, Barberry Bark – Crystal Star Herbs available at Health Food Stores or visit: HealthyHealing.com

---

*Excerpts from "Healthy Healing" – by Linda Page

Dr. Sinatra's Healthy Heart Program*

Dr. Stephen Sinatra strongly believes that the more efficient your body's cells are at creating and burning energy, the better your overall health will be. This is especially true of the heart, which uses more energy than any other organ in the body.

TOP 12 TIPS FOR A HEALTHY HEART

1. **Get on the modified healthy Mediterranean Diet.** I recommend this diet because it offers a combination of healthy fats, moderate protein and fewer carbohydrates – the optimal recipe for heart health. This diet is also rich in alpha-linolenic acid and omega-3 oils, which help prevent blood clotting, reduce blood pressure and prevent cholesterol buildup (see more on page 244).

2. **Raise your fitness level.** I can't think of another lifestyle change with such immediate and long-lasting benefits for your well-being. Even simple exercises strengthen your heart and circulatory system, build stamina and improve your state of mind! The best exercise is the one you will stick with. Walking and dancing are both great and enjoyable. Remember you don't have to work up a sweat or push yourself until you're out of breath.

   I wholeheartedly endorse adding weight-lifting to your exercise regimen to promote a healthy heart and bones. Not only does strength training increase endurance, it can promote healthy blood pressure and improve cholesterol levels and enhance your sense of well-being.

3. **Reduce your stress.** There are many effective stress-reduction techniques, such as: yoga, massage, prayer, visualization, deep breathing exercises, positive affirmations, listening to classical music and meditating or sitting quietly for 15 minutes a day.

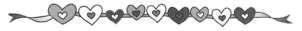

DANCING HELPS YOUR HEART:
A recent study has found that dancing has the same benefit for heart patients as working out at the gym. "Hit the dance floor and help your heart."
– ReadersDigest.com.

*****See more from Dr. Sinatra - excerpts on web: HeartMDinstitute.com*

4. **Take a multi-vitamin** that includes carotenoids, flavonoids, vitamins C, E and B and selenium.

5. **Co-Q10 Ubiquinol** is another strong must. It's one of the best nutrients for promoting heart health.

6. **L-Carnitine**, a nutrient that helps preserve heart health. Take 500mg to 2 grams daily.

7. **Magnesium and Calcium** promote healthy blood pressure and help regulate heart health. Calcium with magnesium, promotes healthy blood vessels. Take daily together 500mg of magnesium and 1,000mg of calcium.

8. **Fish oil** is one of the best sources of healthy fat around. You can eat cold-water fish like salmon and mackerel or take fish or flax oil at least twice a week and/or take a daily fish/flax oil supplement.

9. **Smoking: Stop it!** Research shows that smokers are twice as likely to have serious heart problems.

10. **L-Arginine**, an amino acid that improves blood flow to the heart. Take 2 to 4 grams 2 hours before bedtime.

11. **Nattokinase** is an enzyme and very effective in breaking down fibrin which in turn helps keep blood free-flowing.

12. **Alcohol: Limit it!** One glass of organic red wine daily with dinner is fine, if desired, but hard alcohol is out!

Dr. Sinatra's Modified Mediterranean Diet*

After a great deal of research, I've concluded that the **best overall diet is the Modified, Mediterranean Diet.** This diet can support and balance blood sugar and insulin levels, while giving you more energy and help you find ideal weight or body mass. This diet consists of:

• **Whole grains, raw nuts, seeds, soybeans and legumes** are the basic foundation. These foods provide complex carbohydrates, fiber, protein, vitamins and minerals. Complex carbohydrates are the "slow burners" – they convert to glucose slowly, support stable blood sugar levels, and don't convert to fat as easily as refined carbohydrates.

*See more from Dr. Sinatra - excerpts on web: HeartMDinstitute.com

244

I recommend 1-2 small servings of organic whole grains and 1-2 servings of legumes daily. Finally, 2-3 servings of raw nuts and seeds daily.

• **Fruits** have lots of water, fiber, antioxidants and vitamins and minerals. So, fill up on a delicious healthy fruit bowl! I recommend 1-2 servings of organic fresh fruit daily.

• **Vegetables** make preparing a more nutritious, delicious, inexpensive meal easy and healthy. There are many organic vegetables to choose from. They are full of healthy nutrients and fiber. Use vegetables liberally to make great raw finger snacks, sandwiches and side dishes. I recommend 3-5 servings of organic fresh vegetables daily.

• **High-quality fats** – include olives and olive oil, fatty fish, raw nuts, nut butters, flaxseed, and avocados. I recommend 5-6 servings of healthy fats and oils daily.

• **Fish and eggs** are both important components. Both contain protein and essential fatty acids (EFAs). The right fish has health-boosting benefits. I feel strongly that you should choose toxic-free, migratory cold-water, fatty fish over meat and poultry as often as possible. I recommend 2-3 servings of wild (not farm-raised) fish weekly. Free-range eggs supply essential antioxidants. I recommend 3-6 a week.

• **Organic Dairy products** contain health-promoting calcium, protein, and vitamins B12 and D. I recommend no more than 2 servings per day and only organic!

• **Poultry/Beef/Lamb:** eat in moderation 2-3 servings per week and just 1 serving per week or every other week of beef or lamb *(be sure it is organic, grass fed and hormone-free)*.

Key Benefits of Mediterranean Diet:
Excerpts from: *www.HeartMDinstitute.com*

• High in healthy antioxidants
• More fish, less beef and less dairy
• High in heart healthy olive oil
• Helps normalize your weight
• Higher energy levels and helps fight diseases
• Prevents blood clots, reduces blood pressure
   and helps prevent cholesterol build-up
• Can support and balance blood sugar levels
• High levels of healthy omega-3 fatty acids

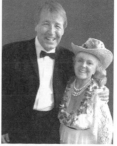

Dr. Sinatra with Patricia

Healthier lifestyle habits can help you reduce your risk for a heart attack. Even simple small changes can make a big difference in your living a healthier, better life.

"Life's Simple 7" can help add years to your life:

1. Maintain a healthy weight
2. Engage in regular exercise
3. Eat a healthy diet
4. Keep blood sugar or glucose at healthy level
5. Manage blood pressure
6. Don't Smoke
7. Manage cholesterol

A healthy diet is one of your most powerful weapons in the fight against heart disease. Be sure to buy and eat plenty of organic fresh fruits and vegetables. Watch out for the saturated and/or partially hydrogenated fats hidden in bakery goods, casseroles, desserts and other foods. If desired have one serving of grilled or baked fish twice a week. Select more meat substitutes such as dried beans, peas, lentils and tofu and use them as entrees or in salads and soups. Raw nuts and seeds, are a good source of protein. Choose organic whole-grain, high-fiber breads.

Exercise more: swimming, cycling, jogging, skiing, aerobic dancing, walking or many other activities can help your heart. Whether it's included in a structured exercise program or part of your daily routine, all physical activity adds up to a healthier heart.

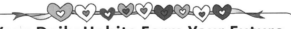

Your Daily Habits Form Your Future

Habits can be wrong or right, good or bad, healthy or unhealthy, rewarding or unrewarding. The right or wrong habits, decisions, actions, words or deeds . . . are up to you! Wisely choose your habits, as they can make or break your life! – Patricia Bragg, Health Crusader

Health is the most natural thing in the world. It is natural to be healthy because we are a part of Mother Nature – we are nature. Nature is trying hard to keep us well, because she needs us in her business.
– Elbert G. Hubbard, American writer, artist and philosopher, 1856-1915

The body and mind are so closely connected that not even a single word or thought can come into existence without being reflected in the personality & health of the individual. – John Holmes Prentiss, 1784-1861

Chapter 24

Healthy Alternative Therapies
and Massage Techniques

Try Them – They Are Working Miracles!

Explore these wonderful natural methods of healing your body. Over 600 Medical Schools in the U.S. are teaching Healthy Alternative Therapies. Please check their websites. Seek and choose the best healing techniques for you:

ACUPUNCTURE / ACUPRESSURE: Acupuncture directs and rechannels body energy by inserting hair-thin needles (use only disposable needles) at specific points on the body. It's used for pain, backaches, migraines and general health and body dysfunctions. Used in Asia for centuries, acupuncture is safe, virtually painless and has no side effects! Acupressure is based on the same principles and uses finger pressure and massage rather than needles. Check web: *AcupunctureToday.com*

CHIROPRACTIC: was founded in Davenport, Iowa in 1885 by Daniel David Palmer. There are now many schools in the U.S., and graduates are joining Health Practitioners in all nations of the world to share healing techniques. Chiropractic is popular and the largest U.S. healing profession benefitting literally millions! Treatment involves soft tissue, spinal and body adjustment to free nervous system of any interferences with normal body functions. Its concern is the functional integrity of the musculoskeletal system. In addition to manual methods, chiropractors use physical therapy modalities, exercise, health and nutritional guidance. Web: *ChiroWeb.com*

247

COLON HYDROTHERAPY: is a safe and effective practice for supporting detoxification, and improving health and vitality. Contact I-ACT (Int'l Association Colon Hydrotherapy) for a certified colon Hydro-Therapist in your area. Web: *i-act.org*

SKIN BRUSHING: daily is wonderful for circulation, toning, cleansing and healing. Use a dry vegetable brush (never nylon) and brush lightly. Helps purify lymph so it's able to detoxify your blood and tissues. Removes old skin cells, uric acid crystals and toxic wastes that come up through skin's pores. Use loofah sponge for variety in shower or tub.

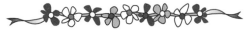

Skin is often called your third kidney because it eliminates toxins from body.

HOMEOPATHY: In 1796, Dr. Samuel Hahnemann, a German physician, developed homeopathy. Patients are treated with "micro" doses of remedies found in nature to trigger the body's own defenses. This homeopathic principle is a safe and nontoxic remedy and is the #1 alternative therapy in Europe and Britain because it is inexpensive, seldom has any side effects, and usually brings fast results. Web: *HomeopathyCenter.org*

NATUROPATHY: Brought to America by Dr. Benedict Lust, M.D., this treatment uses diet, herbs, homeopathy, fasting, exercise, hydrotherapy, manipulation and sunlight. Practitioners work with your body to restore health naturally. They reject surgery and drugs except as a last resort. Web: *www.Naturopathic.org*

OSTEOPATHY: The first School of Osteopathy was founded in 1892 by Dr. Andrew Taylor Still, M.D. There are now 30 U.S. colleges. Treatment involves soft tissue, spinal and body adjustments that free the nervous system from interferences that can cause illness. Healing by adjustment also includes good nutrition, physical therapies, proper breathing and good posture. Dr. Still's premise: if the body structure is altered or abnormal, then proper body function is altered and can cause pain and illness. Web: *www.AcademyofOsteopathy.org*

248

REFLEXOLOGY/ZONE THERAPY: Founded by Eunice Ingham, author of *Stories The Feet Can Tell*, inspired by a Bragg Health Crusade when she was 17. Reflexology helps the body and organs by removing crystalline deposits from reflex areas (nerve endings) of feet and hands through deep pressure massage. Primitive reflexology originated in China and Egypt and Native American Indians and Kenyans self-practiced it for centuries. Reflexology activates body's flow of healing and energy by dislodging deposits. Visit Eunice Ingham and nephew Dwight Byer's website: *www.Reflexology-usa.net*

WATER THERAPY: Soothing detox shower: apply organic olive oil to skin, alternate hot and cold water, every 2-3 minutes. Massage body while under hot, filtered spray. Garden hose massage is great in summer or anytime. Hot detox soak bath (diabetics use warm water) 20 minutes with cup of Epsom salts or apple cider vinegar. This soak helps pull out the toxins by creating an artificial fever cleanse.

Time waits for no one, treasure and protect every moment you have!

To live is to know what counts and is important in your life. – Martin Grey

Alternative Health Therapies & Massage Techniques

ALEXANDER TECHNIQUE: helps end improper use of neuromuscular system, helps bring body posture into balance. Eliminates psycho-physical interferences, helps release long-held tension, and aids in re-establishing muscle tone. For more info see web: *AlexanderTechnique.com*

FELDENKRAIS METHOD: Dr. Moshe Feldenkrais founded this in the late 1940s. This Method leads to improved posture and helps create ease and more efficiency of body movement. This Method is a great stress removal. Web: *Feldenkrais.com*

REIKI: A Japanese form of massage that means "Universal Life Energy." Reiki Massage helps the body to detoxify, then re-balance and heal itself. Discovered in the ancient Sutra manuscripts by Dr. Mikao Usui in Japan 1922. Web: *Reiki.org*

ROLFING: Developed by Ida Rolf in the 1930's in the U.S. Rolfing is also called structural processing and postural release, or structural dynamics. It is based on the concept that distortions (accidents, injuries, falls, etc.) and the effects of gravity on the body cause upsets and long-term stress in the body. Rolfing helps to achieve balance and improved body posture. Methods involve the use of stretching, with gentle deep tissue massage and relaxation techniques to loosen old injuries, break bad movement and posture patterns. Web: *Rolf.org*

TRAGERING: Founded by Dr. Milton Trager M.D., who was inspired at age 18 by Paul C. Bragg to become a doctor. It is a mind-body learning method that involves gentle shaking and rocking, allowing the body to let go, releasing tensions and lengthening the muscles for more body peace and health. Tragering can do miracle healing where needed in the body frame, muscles and the entire body. Web: *Trager.com*

MASSAGE & AROMATHERAPY: works two ways: the essence (aroma) relaxes, as does healing massages. Essential oils are extracted from flowers, leaves, roots, seeds and barks. These are usually massaged into skin, inhaled or used in a bath to help the body relax, soothe and heal. The oils, used for centuries to treat numerous ailments, are revitalizing and energizing for the body and mind. Example: Tiger balm, MSM, echinacea and arnica help relieve muscle aches. (Avoid skin creams and lotions with mineral oil – it clogs the skin's pores.) Use these natural oils for the skin: almond, avocado, use organic olive oil and mix with aromatic essential oils: rosemary, lavender, rose, jasmine, sandalwood or lemon-balm, etc. – 6 oz. oil and 4 drops of an essential oil. Web: *www.Aromatherapy.com*

Alternative Health Therapies & Massage Techniques

MASSAGE – SELF: Paul C. Bragg often said, *"You can be your own best massage therapist, even if you have only one good hand."* Near-miraculous health improvements have been achieved by victims of accidents or strokes in bringing life back to afflicted parts of their own bodies by self-massage and even vibrators. Treatments can be day or night, almost continual. Self-massage also helps achieve relaxation at day's end. Families and friends can learn and exchange massages; it's a wonderful sharing experience. Remember, babies love and thrive with daily massages, start from birth. Family pets also love soothing, healing touch of massages. Web: *RD.com/health/wellness/learn-the-art-of-self-massage*

MASSAGE – SHIATSU: Japanese massage form applies pressure from fingers, hands, elbows and even knees along the same points as acupuncture. Shiatsu originated in Japan and is based on traditional Chinese medicine, and has been widely practiced around the world since 1970s. Shiatsu has been used in Asia for centuries to relieve pain, common ills, muscle stress and to aid lymphatic circulation. See web: *centerpointmn.com/the-benefits-of-shiatsu-massage*

250 *MASSAGE – SWEDISH:* One of the oldest and the most popular and widely used massage techniques. This deep body massage soothes and promotes healthy circulation and is a great way to loosen and relax tight muscles before and after exercise. See web: *www.MassageDen.com/swedish-massage.shtml*

MASSAGE – SPORTS: An important health support system for professional and amateur athletes. Sports massage improves circulation and mobility to injured tissue, enables athletes to recover more rapidly from myofascial injury, reduces muscle soreness and chronic strain patterns. Soft tissues are freed of trigger points and adhesions, thus contributing to improvement of peak neuromuscular functioning and athletic performance.

Author's Comment: We have personally sampled many of these Alternative Therapies. It's estimated America's health care costs are over $2.6 trillion. It's more important than ever to be responsible for our own health! This includes seeking dedicated holistic health practitioners to keep us well by inspiring us to practice prevention! These Alternative Healing Therapies are also popular and getting results: aromatherapy, Ayurvedic, biofeedback, guided imagery, herbs, hyperbaric oxygen, music, meditation, magnets, saunas, tai chi, Qi gong, Pilates, Rebounder, yoga, etc. Explore them and be open to improving your earthly temple for a healthy, happier, longer life.

Seek and find the best for your body, mind and soul. – Patricia Bragg

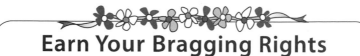

Earn Your Bragging Rights
Live The Bragg Healthy Lifestyle
To Attain Supreme Physical, Mental,
Emotional and Spiritual Health!

With your new awareness, understanding and sincere commitment of how to live The Bragg Healthy Lifestyle!

God bless you and your family and may He give you the strength, the courage and the patience to win your battle to re-enter the Healthy Garden of Eden while you are still living here on Earth with more years to enjoy it all!

With Blessings of Health, Peace, Joy and Love,

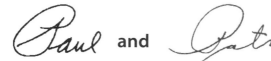

Paul and *Patricia*

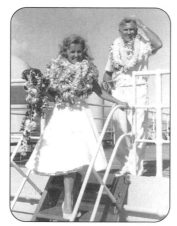

*Health Crusaders
Paul C. Bragg and
daughter Patricia
traveled the
world spreading
health, inspiring
millions to renew
and revitalize
their health.*

251

*The Bragg books are written to inspire and guide you to health,
fitness and longevity. Remember, the book you don't read won't help.
So please reread Bragg Books and live The Bragg Healthy Lifestyle
to enjoy a healthy fulfilled life!*

---

*I never suspected that I would have to learn how to live –
that there were specific disciplines and ways of seeing the world
that I had to master before I could awaken to a simple,
healthy, happy, uncomplicated life.– Dan Millman, author
"The Way of the Peaceful Warrior" • peacefulwarrior.com
A Bragg fan and admirer since his Stanford University coaching days.*

---

*A truly good book teaches me better than to just read it,
I must soon lay it down and commence living in its wisdom.
What I began by reading, I must finish by acting! – Henry David Thoreau*

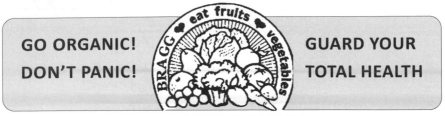

GO ORGANIC! DON'T PANIC! — eat fruits • vegetables — BRAGG — **GUARD YOUR TOTAL HEALTH**

FROM THE AUTHORS

This book was written for YOU! It can be your passport to a healthy, long, vital life. We in the Alternative Health Therapies join hands in one common objective – promoting a high standard of health for everyone. Healthy nutrition points the way – which is Mother Nature and God's way. This book teaches you how to work with them, not against them! Health doctors, therapists, nurses, teachers and caregivers are becoming more dedicated than ever before to keeping their patients healthy and fit. This book was written to emphasize the great needed importance of healthy lifestyle living for health and longevity, close to Mother Nature and God.

Statements in this book are scientific health findings, known facts of physiology and biological therapeutics. Paul C. Bragg practiced natural methods of living for over 80 years with highly beneficial results, knowing that they were safe and of great value. His daughter Patricia lectured and co-authored the Bragg Health Books with him and continues carrying on the Bragg Healthy Lifestyle.

Paul C. Bragg and daughter Patricia express their opinions solely as public health educators. They offer no cure for disease. Only the body has the ability to cure a person. Experts may disagree with some of the statements made in this book. However, such statements are considered to be factual, based on the long-time experience of dedicated pioneer health crusaders Paul C. Bragg and Patricia Bragg. If you suspect you have a medical problem, please always seek qualified health care professionals to help you make the healthiest, wisest and best-informed choices!

Count your blessings daily while you do your 30-to 45-minute brisk walks and exercises with these affirmations – health! strength! youth! vitality! peace! laughter! humility! understanding! forgiveness! joy! and love for eternity! and soon all these qualities will come flooding and bouncing into your life. With blessings of super health, peace and love to you, our dear friends – our readers. – Patricia Bragg, Health Crusader

Oxygen is the main nutrient of the body. When we improve our oxygen intake, we enhance our immune system and the body's ability to detoxify and stay healthy for a long life. – Dr. Michael Schachter, Columbia University

If I were to name the three most precious resources of life, I would say books, friends and nature; and the greatest of these, at least the most constant and always at hand is Mother Nature and God. – John Burroughs

```
□□□□□□□□□□□□□□□□□□□□□□□□□□□□□□□□
```
BRAGG PHOTO GALLERY
```
□□□□□□□□□□□□□□□□□□□□□□□□□□□□□□□□
```

PATRICIA & PAUL C. BRAGG, N.D., Ph.D.
Dynamic Daughter & Father are World Health Crusaders

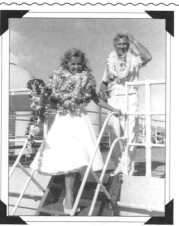

BRAGG PRODUCTS
HEALTH IS HERE

During the past century, Bragg Live Food Products developed and pioneered the very first line of Health Foods, from vitamins and minerals to organic nuts, seeds, and sun-dried fruits. This included over 365 health products, – *"one for each day of the year!"* says daughter Patricia Bragg.

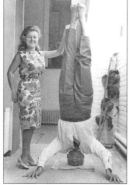

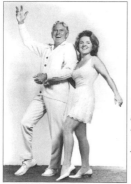

"You have recharged me with joy, hope, love and encouragement, which poured from your words. I am now fasting and using ACV. You have certainly improved my life!"
– Marie Furia, New Jersey

Patricia and father, Paul
on world trip in 1950's,
during stop in Tahiti.

"Thanks for The Bragg Healthy Lifestyle that you shared with me and you are sharing with millions of others worldwide."
– John Gray, Ph.D., author

Picture from
People Magazine August, 1975.

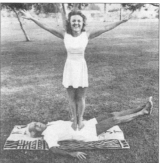

Patricia Bragg stands on her father's stomach. Paul's stomach muscles are so strong he can lift Patricia up and down!

253

PAUL C. BRAGG, N.D., Ph.D.
HEALTH CRUSADER
Life Extension Specialist and Originator of Health Food Stores

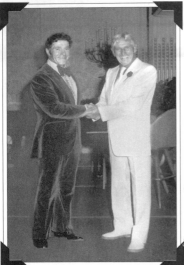

I have experienced a beautiful, remarkable, spiritual and physical awakening since reading Bragg Health Books. I'll never be the same again.
– Sandy Tuttle, Ohio

With every new day comes new strength and new thoughts.
– Eleanor Roosevelt

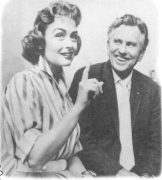

Actress Donna Reed saying "Health First" with Paul C. Bragg.

Dr. Paul C. Bragg (right) Creator Health Food Stores, Pioneer Life Extension Specialist, with his prize student Jack LaLanne. Paul started him on the royal road to health over 85 years ago!

Paul C. Bragg spent much of his time at the Hollywood Studios meeting with top Stars and motion picture industry executives, giving health lectures and private consultations. Dr. Paul C. Bragg was Hollywood's first highly respected, health, fitness and nutrition advisor to the Stars.

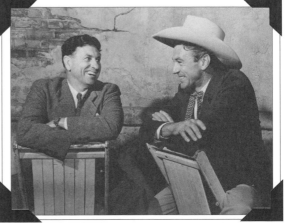

Paul C. Bragg with Gary Cooper, famous American film actor, best known for his many Western films.

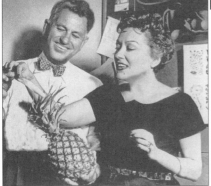

Paul C. Bragg with the famous Hollywood Actress Gloria Swanson, who was leading star in 20s, 30s and 40s. Gloria became a Bragg Health Devotee at 18 and she often would Health Crusade with Bragg during the 1950s.

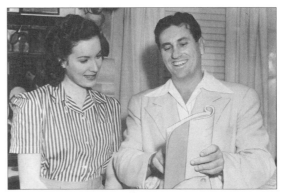

Maureen O'Hara and Paul C. Bragg. This Irish film actress and singer was best noted for playing in "Miracle on 34th Street" and "The Quiet Man."

PAUL C. BRAGG, N.D., Ph.D. STAYING HEALTHY & FIT

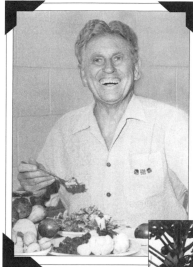

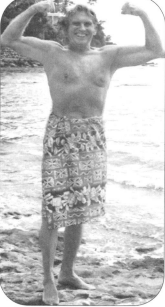

I'd like to thank you for teaching me how to take control of my health! I lost 55 pounds and I feel "great!" Bragg books have showed me vitality, happiness and being close to Mother Nature. You both are real "Crusaders for Health for the World." Thanks!
– Leonard Amato

Dr. Paul C. Bragg and daughter Patricia were my early guiding inspiration to my health career.
– Jeffery Bland, Ph.D., Famous Food Scientist

Paul C. Bragg owes his powerful body and superb health to living exclusively on live, vital, healthy, organic rich foods.

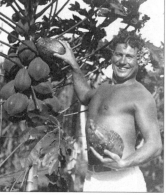

❀ **The best thing about the future is that it only comes one day at a time.** ❀
– Abraham Lincoln

Paul C. Bragg in Tahiti 1920's gathering tropical papaya fruit.

Dear Friends – you cannot know how greatly you have impacted my life and some of my friends! We love your Bragg Health Books, teachings and products and are now living healthier, happier lives. Thanks!
– Winnie Brown, Arizona

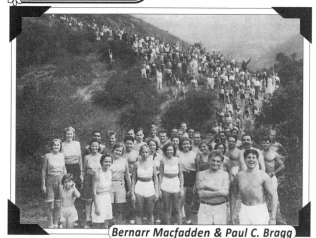

Bernarr Macfadden & Paul C. Bragg

A thousand happy Bragg Health Students enjoy hiking, exercise and fresh air on the trail to Mount Hollywood (above Griffith Observatory) in beautiful California, summer of 1932.

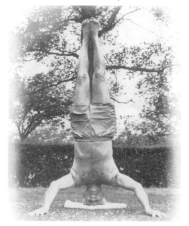

Paul C. Bragg exercising Regent's Park, London.

PHOTO GALLERY
PAUL & PATRICIA BRAGG

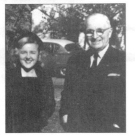

Patricia with 33rd President Harry S. Truman at his home in Independence, Missouri.

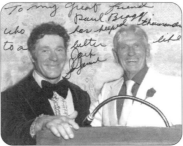

Paul C. Bragg, Creator of Health Food Stores, with his prize student Jack LaLanne, who thanks Bragg for saving his life at 15.

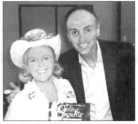

Patrica Bragg with Dr. Jeffrey Smith. He is leader in getting GMO's out of US foods. See GMO video by Jeffrey Smith and narrated by Lisa Oz (Dr. Oz's wife) on web: *GeneticRouletteMovie.com*

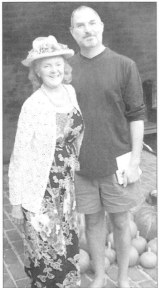

Patricia visiting with Steve Jobs at his home in Palo Alto during the Thanksgiving Holidays.

"I've been reading Bragg Books since high school. I'm thankful for the Bragg Healthy Lifestyle and admire their Health Crusading for a healthier, happier world." – Steve Jobs, Creator – Apple Computer

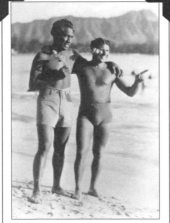

Paul in 1920 with his swimming & surfing friend, Duke Kahanamoku, Waikiki Beach, Diamond Head.

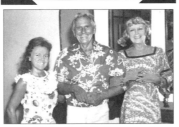

Patricia, Paul C. Bragg and Mrs. Duke (Nadine) Kahanamoku. (Nadine is Patricia's Godmother).

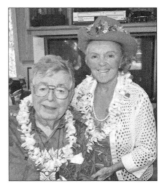

Dr. Earl Bakken with Patricia. He's famous for inventing the first Transistor Pacemaker. His firm Medtronic, developed it and a Resuscitator for fixing ailing hearts that have and are saving thousands of lives. Dr. Bakken lived in Hawaii.

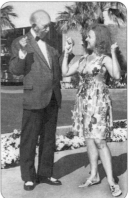

"I cannot remember a time when the Golden Rule was not my motto and precept, the torch that guided my footsteps."* – J.C. Penney

J.C.Penney & Patricia → exercising. They walked often in Palm Springs when he and his wife visited in the winter to enjoy the warm desert sunshine.

*The Golden Rule: Do unto others as you would have them do unto you.

HEALTH CRUSADING TO HOLLYWOOD STARS

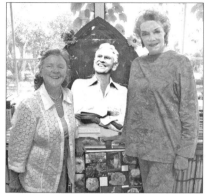

Patricia with friend Actress Jane Russell. Famous Hollywood Star of 40s to 60s.

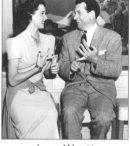

Jane Wyatt learning about health with Paul C. Bragg.

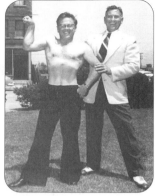

Mickey Rooney with Paul. Rooney was an American film actor and entertainer. He won multiple awards and had one of the longest careers of any actor to age 93!

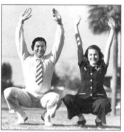

Paul C. Bragg exercising with Actress Helen Parrish.

"Thank you Paul & Patricia Bragg for my simple, easy-to-follow Healthy Lifestyle. You make my days healthy!" – Clint Eastwood, Academy Award Winning Film Producer, Director, Actor and Bragg follower for over 65 years.

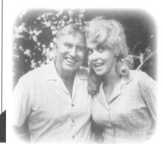

Paul C. Bragg and Donna Douglas, one of Hollywood's most beautiful and talented health advocates. She played the part of "Elly-May" in the *Beverly Hillbillies*, which became one of the longest-running series in television history and was the #1 show in America in its first 2 years.

> ❀ **Life is a Miracle Minute by Minute Year by Year!** ❀

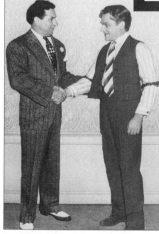

Paul C. Bragg with James Cagney, American film actor. He won major awards for wide variety of roles. The American Film Institute ranked Cagney 8th among the Greatest Male Hollywood Stars of All Time.

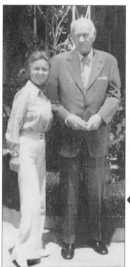

Patricia with Conrad Hilton

← Hotel founder, Conrad Hilton with Patricia Bragg, his Healthy Lifestyle Teacher. *"I wouldn't be alive today if it wasn't for the Braggs and their Bragg Healthy Lifestyle!"* – Conrad Hilton

"Thank you for your website. What a wealth of info to learn about how to live and eat healthy. Many Blessings!" – Michel & Mary, California

PHOTO GALLERY
PAUL C. BRAGG, N.D., Ph.D.
PROMOTES HEALTH & FITNESS!

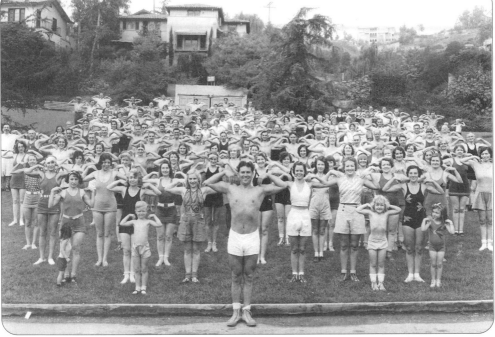

Paul C. Bragg leading an exercise class in Griffith Park, Hollywood, CA – circa 1920s.

Bragg Healthy Lifestyle works Miracles! – Jack LaLanne

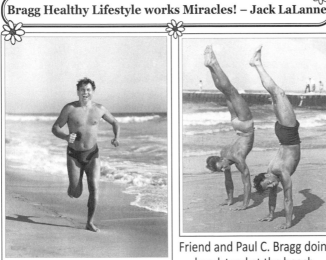

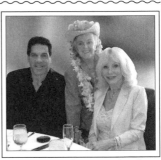

Patricia with Lou and wife Carla at Elaine LaLanne's 90th Birthday Party.

Friend and Paul C. Bragg doing handstand at the beach.

Paul running on Coney Island, New York, where he was a member of the Coney Island Polar Bear Club, known for Cold Water Swimming, 1930s.

TV Hulk Actor Lou Ferrigno gives thanks to Bragg Books. Lou went from puny to become Super Hulk! ➤

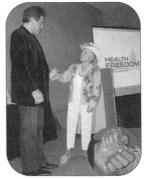

"I lost 102 lbs. with The Bragg Healthy Lifestyle and I have kept it off for over 15 years, staying away from white flour, sugar and other processed foods."
– Dee McCaffrey, Chemist & Diet Counselor, Tempe, AZ

Lou & Patricia in Chicago Health Freedom Expo.

PATRICIA CONTINUING BRAGG HEALTH CRUSADE!

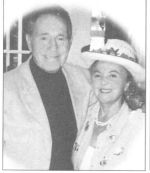
Jack LaLanne with Patricia.

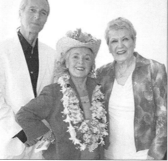
Jon & Elaine LaLanne with Patricia.

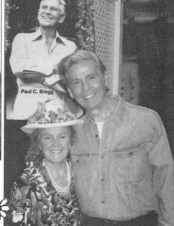

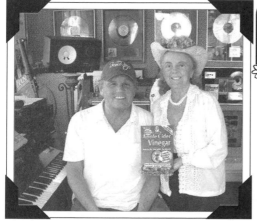
Patricia in studio with famous Beach Boy Bruce Johnston, Bragg follower over 40 years. He played for her their latest records.

Mother Nature Loves US!

Patricia Bragg with Bill Galt inspired by Bragg Books, he founded Good Earth Restaurants.

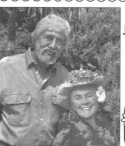
Patricia with Jean-Michel Cousteau Ocean Explorer & Environmentalist. OceanFutures.org

Enjoy a Lifetime of Radiant Health

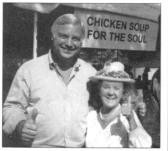
Patricia with Jack Canfield, Bragg follower, Motivational Speaker and Co-Producer of *Chicken Soup For The Soul.*

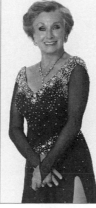

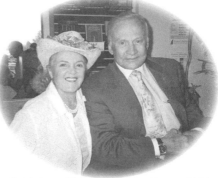
Patricia with Astronaut Buzz Aldrin, celebrating over 50 years since pilot of Apollo 11 first landed on the moon.

Famous Hollywood Actress Cloris Leachman, ardent health follower who sparkled with health and vitality said, *"The Miracle of Fasting Book is a miracle . . . it cured my asthma, my years of arthritis and many other health problems. I praise Paul and Patricia daily for their Health Crusading!"*

259

PAUL & PATRICIA BRAGG
HEALTH CRUSADING

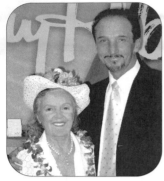

Patricia with Jay Robb.

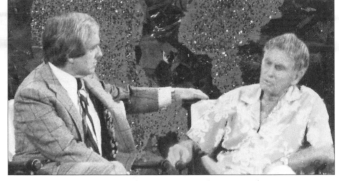

Paul C. Bragg on the Merv Griffin Show, 1976.

Paul Bragg inspired me many years ago with The Miracle of Fasting Book and his pioneering philosophy on health. His daughter Patricia is a testament to the ageless value of living The Bragg Healthy Lifestyle. – Jay Robb, author of The Fruit Flush

During the many years Patricia worked with her father, she was right beside him, assisting him on Bragg Health Crusades worldwide. They were a great team, when you looked at them, you would see only two people headed in the same healthy direction!

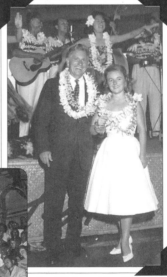

I am a big fan of Paul Bragg. I fast and follow The Bragg Healthy Lifestyle daily. The world and I are blessed with the health teachings of Paul and Patricia Bragg!
– Tony Robbins • TonyRobbins.com

❀ **Dream big, think big and enjoy the many miracles.** ❀

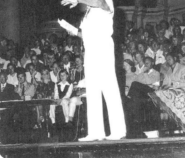

Paul & Daughter Patricia, Royal Hawaiian, Honolulu.

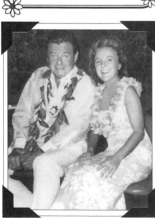

Paul – London Bragg Health Crusade.

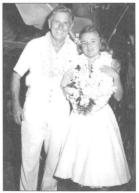

Actor Arthur Godfrey with Patricia, in Honolulu celebrating his 79th birthday.

Health Crusaders Paul C. Bragg and daughter Patricia traveled the world spreading health, inspiring millions to renew and revitalize their health.
Bragg Mottos:
3 John 2 and Genesis 6:3

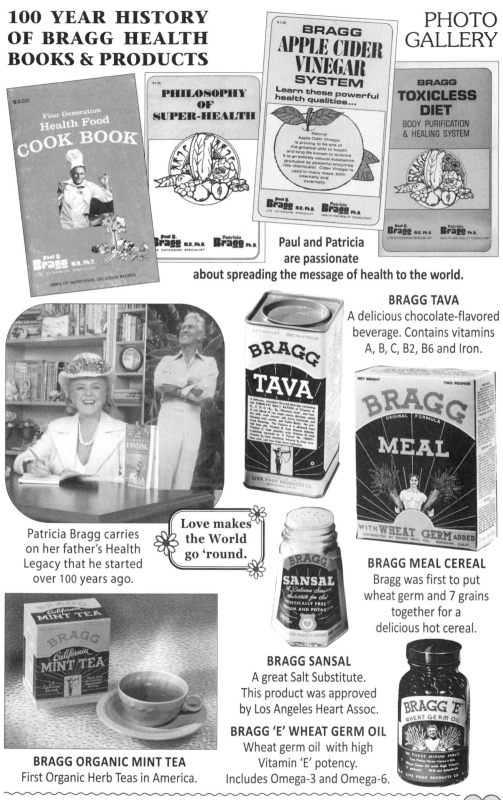

100 YEAR HISTORY OF BRAGG HEALTH BOOKS & PRODUCTS

PHOTO GALLERY

Four Generation Health Food COOK BOOK

PHILOSOPHY OF SUPER-HEALTH

BRAGG APPLE CIDER VINEGAR SYSTEM
Learn these powerful health qualities...

BRAGG TOXICLESS DIET
BODY PURIFICATION & HEALING SYSTEM

Paul and Patricia are passionate about spreading the message of health to the world.

Patricia Bragg carries on her father's Health Legacy that he started over 100 years ago.

Love makes the World go 'round.

BRAGG TAVA
A delicious chocolate-flavored beverage. Contains vitamins A, B, C, B2, B6 and Iron.

BRAGG MEAL CEREAL
Bragg was first to put wheat germ and 7 grains together for a delicious hot cereal.

BRAGG SANSAL
A great Salt Substitute. This product was approved by Los Angeles Heart Assoc.

BRAGG 'E' WHEAT GERM OIL
Wheat germ oil with high Vitamin 'E' potency. Includes Omega-3 and Omega-6.

BRAGG ORGANIC MINT TEA
First Organic Herb Teas in America.

"Our lives have completely turned around! Our family is feeling so healthy, we must tell you about it."– Gene & Joan Zollner, parents of 11, Washington

261

PHOTO GALLERY — Celebrating Years of Health Crusading

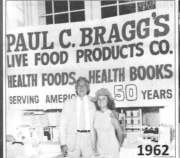

HALL of LEGENDS
Patricia Bragg

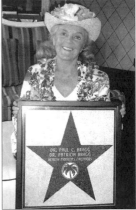

1962

Paul C. Bragg with Patricia, celebrating over 50 years of Bragg Health Products, Books & Crusading worldwide, spreading Health around the world.

"Palm Spring Walk of Stars" – Patricia with Bragg Star.

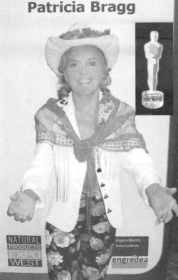

Natural Foods Expo in Anaheim with 65,000 attendees from around the world honored Patricia Bragg and her father Paul C. Bragg as treasured Health Food Industry Legends.

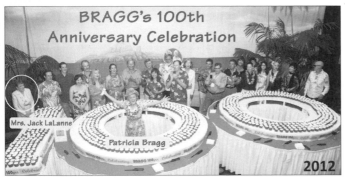

BRAGG's 100th Anniversary Celebration

Mrs. Jack LaLanne

Patricia Bragg

2012

Patricia, Staff & 1,000 Friends celebrated our 100 years of Bragg Healthy Products, Books & Health Crusading! We are proud Pioneers in this Big Health Industry that is helping to keep the world healthier! With Blessings of Health, Peace & Love to You!

Patricia

100 Year Anniversary Party celebrated at the Natural Foods Expo in Anaheim

Bragg Hawaii Exercise Class was founded by Worldwide Health Crusader and Fitness Legend, Dr. Paul C. Bragg. He wanted to create a dynamic, Free Community Exercise Class, and he often taught these classes himself for many years. Patricia Bragg continues her father's health legacy by supporting the Bragg Exercise Class and participates in the class whenever she is in Hawaii.

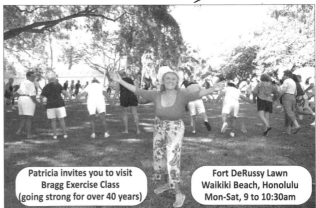

Patricia invites you to visit Bragg Exercise Class (going strong for over 40 years)

Fort DeRussy Lawn Waikiki Beach, Honolulu Mon-Sat, 9 to 10:30am

"Please make a record of your family history & background. Take pictures – make your own 'Photo Gallery'. Take videos – make movies of your children, spouse, mother and father, family gatherings, etc. These memories are precious & important to save for future generations." – Patricia Bragg

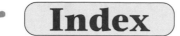

Index

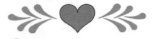 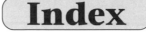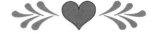

Dream big, think big, but enjoy the small miracles of everyday life!

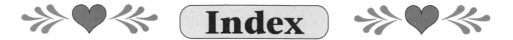

Love, kindness and compassion are necessities, not luxuries . . .
without them humanity cannot survive. – The Dalai Lama

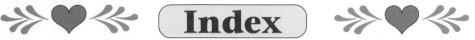

Healthy Mind Habit: Wake up and say, "Today I am going to be happier, healthier and wiser in my daily living! I am the captain of my life and am going to steer it to living a 100% healthy lifestyle!" Fact is happy people look younger and have fewer health problems! – Patricia Bragg, Pioneer Health Crusader

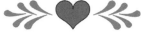
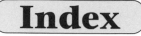 **Index**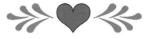

Roses are God's autograph of beauty, fragrance and love.
– Paul C. Bragg, ND, PhD.

Through our actions and deeds, rather than promises, let us display
the essence of love – perfect harmony in motion! – Philip Glyn, Welsh Poet

A book is a garden, an orchard, a storehouse, a party, a mentor,
a teacher, a guidepost, a counsellor. – Henry Ward Beecher

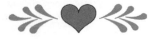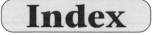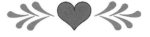

Index

May your mind forever sparkle like a star, your heart remain pure as new fallen snow and your spirit forever sense the wonderment of a child. – Mary Summer Rain

Peace is not a season, it is a way of life.

Apple Cider Vinegar - Miracle Health System

BY PAUL C. BRAGG, N.D., PH.D.
and PATRICIA BRAGG

Paul C. Bragg, originator of health stores in America, and world-renowned health crusader Patricia Bragg, introduced America to the life-changing value of Apple Cider Vinegar, with the miracle enzyme known as "the mother." Now a widely popular beverage, this book reveals the legendary health-and life-giving versatility of apple cider vinegar. Following in the footsteps of Hippocrates, who taught the benefits of ACV to his patients in 400 BC, the Braggs teach dozens of reasons to use vinegar, including as a beauty aid, for skin treatments, in recipes, as an antibiotic, anti-septic, hair-revitalizing rinse, headache reliever, and weight reducer. ACV optimizes digestive health and can reduce or eliminate acid reflux. Paul and Patricia Bragg have helped millions heal and restore their vitality and zest for life through their time-tested understanding of natural health. *Apple Cider Vinegar: Miracle Health System* is informative, entertaining, and invaluable for anyone wanting to feel their best.

Bragg Healthy Lifestyle - Vital Living at Any Age

BY PAUL C. BRAGG, N.D., PH.D.
and PATRICIA BRAGG

Learn the simple strategies of radical health and vibrant wellness that The Bragg Healthy Lifestyle has brought to millions! What is an ageless body? For health pioneers Paul C. Bragg and Patricia Bragg, an ageless body sparkles with vitality, immune strength, mental clarity, and digestive ease. The Braggs teach why a toxic-free diet maximizes energy, supports weight loss, and can help heal illness and disease. In the newly revised *Bragg Healthy Lifestyle: Vital Living At Any Age*, the trailblazing father-daughter team who alerted us nearly a century ago to the dangers of sugar and toxic foods, detail every key aspect of creating and maintaining ageless health, including detoxification, stress-release, nutrition, exercise and the importance of taking charge of not only what goes into our bodies, but practices such as fasting, which release the toxins that may unnecessarily accelerate the aging process. "You are what you eat, drink, breathe, think, say and do," is the Bragg motto. From the foods we eat to our outlook, the environments we live in and even in our physical activities, the authors encourage readers to replace toxins with nutrients, flush out poisons and waste efficiently, exercise, breathe deeply and well, and cultivate happiness and harmony in our daily lives.

HEALTH SCIENCE
7127 Hollister Avenue, Suite 25A, Box 249, Santa Barbara, CA 93117
Toll-Free: (833) 408-1122

Building Powerful Nerve Force & Positive Energy - Reduce Stress, Worry and Anger

BY PAUL C. BRAGG, N.D., PH.D.
and PATRICIA BRAGG

What is Nerve Force and why should you care about it? According to mental health trailblazers Paul C. Bragg and Patricia Bragg, "Nerve Force" is a type of life energy stored in the nerves, muscles, organs, and brain. The more Nerve Force you have, the quicker you can re-charge it, and the healthier, happier, and more satisfying a life you will lead. If you suffer from burnout, stress, fatigue, anxiety, insomnia or depression, this book is for you! We know that the ability to feel joy and peace is essential to a complete experience of vitality and wellness. Our thoughts, our attitudes, our outlook, and our emotional well-being are all dependent on having a powerful "Nerve Force." Just like any muscle that we can develop and strengthen, we can build our Nerve Force so that we are resilient, relaxed, and calm, even during times of stress. Paul C. Bragg and Patricia Bragg show you how with simple mental exercises and suggestions for specific foods that replenish your Nerve Force, as well as foods that deplete it, in this newly revised edition of *Building Powerful Nerve Force & Positive Energy* the father-daughter team explains to readers the reward of paying attention to the energy that is responsible for not only our physical capabilities and our vital body functions, but our ability to process information and feel centered and grounded, no matter what life throws at us. They teach us that maintaining a healthy Nerve Force, leads to a balanced and fruitful life.

Super Power Breathing - For Optimum Health & Healing

BY PAUL C. BRAGG, N.D., PH.D.
and PATRICIA BRAGG

Do you sometimes find that you are panting instead of breathing? Many of us do! This can cause headaches, anxiety, fatigue, and brain fog. The quality of our breath determines the quality of our life! This book teaches us how to breathe in a way that replenishes the body with the oxygen it so deeply craves. "The more effectively we breathe, the more effectively we live," write the authors, world-renowned health pioneers Paul C. Bragg and Patricia Bragg. "Super Power Breathing can make your life-force stronger, calmer and smarter." The Super Power Breathing program has been followed by Olympic athletes and millions of Bragg followers, and is filled with simple exercises for energizing and rejuvenating your breath, and your whole body. Research shows that we use only one-fourth to one-half of our lung capacity with each breath. This starves our body much like if we are depriving it of food. We are slowly robbing our body of its most vital, invisible nourishment – oxygen. In its newly revised form, the Bragg Super Power Breathing Program will give you all the tools you need to shift from shallow breathing to taking deep, oxygen-filled, life-giving breaths!

271

Water - The Shocking Truth

BY PAUL C. BRAGG, N.D., PH.D.
and PATRICIA BRAGG

The water you drink can literally make or break your health. The purity of our water is the most critical element in maintaining radical vitality, and healing from illness and disease. In this newly revised edition of *Water: The Shocking Truth*, health crusaders Paul C. Bragg and Patricia Bragg reveal the dangers of tap water, which research shows can be responsible for many ailments, due to the addition of dangerous chemicals such as fluoride and chlorine. In this book, the trailblazing father-daughter team teach the many functions water performs in the body, from regulating the various systems to flushing the body of waste and toxins. But what if the substance we use to cleanse our bodies is itself polluted? With the mandatory fluoridation of water in the municipal water systems, the authors assert that has been the case for decades. Added to the public water supply to prevent tooth decay starting in the 1950s, fluoride has long been known to be a toxin, used in pesticides and rat poisons. Learn what types of water are optimal to drink, how and why to detox your body with nature's most life-giving liquid, and the health-and-life-saving value of installing a water filter in your shower!

Bragg Back & Foot Fitness Program -
Keys to a Pain-Free Back & Strong Healthy Feet

BY PAUL C. BRAGG, N.D., PH.D.
and PATRICIA BRAGG

If you are suffering with back or foot pain, look no further for a comprehensive program that will restore health to the parts of your body that carry you through life! Remember when we were children, and we had the kind of energy and flexibility to play for hours? Agile and active, we could twist, bend, stretch and climb with little effort. However, hours looking at a computer screen, a sedentary lifestyle and poor posture can take their toll. Eventually our backs start to hurt and cramp with every movement, and our feet ache after just a short walk. We start feeling "old." In *Bragg Back & Foot Fitness Program*, the father-daughter team of world-renowned health pioneers, Paul C. Bragg and Patricia Bragg teach how to speed the healing of injuries and develop a strong and flexible back and healthy feet, rejuvenating and re-energizing our bodies in the process. The trailblazing health experts who brought wellness and vitality to millions, including fitness guru Jack LaLanne, outline the keys to a healthy spine, pain-free back and bunion-free feet through nutritional support and clearly illustrated, simple exercises, as well as other tips for posture and massage. Paul and Patricia Bragg reveal the healing properties of herbs, effective ways to practice foot reflexology, how to deal with arthritis, athlete's foot, plantar fasciitis, and foot problems caused by diabetes. By following the authors' Back and Foot Care Program, you can begin to treat your body as Mother Nature intended you to, and creating painless feet, a strong back and a powerful body will begin!

PATRICIA BRAGG
Health Crusader and "Angel of Health and Healing"

Author, Lecturer, Nutritionist, Health & Lifestyle Educator to World Leaders, Hollywood Stars, Singers, Athletes & Millions.

Patricia is a life-long health advocate and activist, admired internationally for her passionate work promoting healthy living. For many years she traveled the world, teaching The Bragg Healthy Lifestyle for physical, spiritual, emotional health and joy. She was invited to give lectures, visited radio shows, was profiled in magazines and appealed to people of all ages, nationalities and walks-of-life. Together with Paul, she co-authored a collection of ten books, with inspiration and techniques for living a long, vital, happy life. Now in her 90s and living on an organic farm in California, Patricia herself is a testament to these teachings and the sparkling symbol of health, perpetual youth and radiant energy.

PAUL C. BRAGG, N.D., Ph.D.
Life Extension Specialist • World Health Crusader
Lecturer and Advisor to Olympic Athletes, Royalty, Stars & Millions.
Originator of Health Food Stores & Founder of Health Movement Worldwide

Paul C. Bragg was at the forefront of the modern health movement, having inspired generations to turn toward wellness. At a young age, Paul turned his own health around by developing an eating, breathing and exercise program to build strength and vitality. From this life-changing experience, he pledged to dedicate the rest of his life to promoting a healthy lifestyle. He opened one of the country's first health food stores, which eventually led to the creation of the Bragg Live Foods company. With a devoted following, Paul traveled giving lectures and sharing his expertise, while serving as an advisor to athletes and movie stars alike. Even Jack LaLanne, the original television fitness guru, credited Paul with having introduced him to the importance of healthy living. In addition to the books Paul wrote with Patricia, they co-hosted television and radio shows and worked together to bring wellness to the world. Paul himself excelled in athletics, loved the ocean and the outdoors, and radiated with health and a warm smile.

Patricia inspires you to Renew, Rejuvenate and Revitalize your Life with "The Bragg Healthy Lifestyle" Books. Millions have benefitted from these life-changing philosophies with a longer, healthier, happier life!

273

Take Time for 12 Things

1. Take time to **Work** –
   it is the price of success.

2. Take time to **Think** –
   it is the source of power.

3. Take time to **Play** –
   it is the secret of youth.

4. Take time to **Read** –
   it is the foundation of knowledge.

5. Take time to **Worship** –
   it is the highway of reverence and
   washes the dust of earth from our eyes.

6. Take time to **Help and Enjoy Friends** –
   it is the source of happiness.

7. Take time to **Love and Share** –
   it is the one sacrament of life.

8. Take time to **Dream** –
   it hitches the soul to the stars.

9. Take time to **Laugh** –
   it is the singing that helps life's loads.

10. Take time for **Beauty** –
    it is everywhere in nature.

11. Take time for **Health** –
    it is the true wealth and treasure of life.

12. Take time to **Plan** –
    it is the secret of being able to have time
    for the first 11 things.

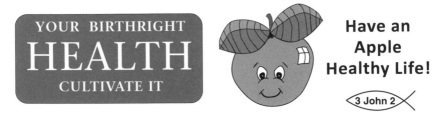

YOUR BIRTHRIGHT

HEALTH

CULTIVATE IT

Have an
Apple
Healthy Life!

3 John 2

*Teach me thy way, LORD, lead me in a straight path,
because of my oppressors. – Psalm 27:11*